#1 WEIGHTLOSS PLAN

30 Day

HEALTHY Eating

Frank A. Kelemen

Contents

7-day healthy meal plan:

To fast-track into a Healthy Eating habit, here is a 7 day meal plan.

Day 1:

- Breakfast: Whole grain cereal with low-fat milk and a banana
- Mid-Morning Snack: A handful of almonds and an apple
- Lunch: Grilled chicken salad with whole grain bread
- Afternoon Snack: Low-fat yogurt with chia seeds
- Dinner: Baked salmon with quinoa and steamed broccoli
- Evening Snack: A pear and a small handful of walnuts

Day 2:

- Breakfast: Oatmeal with low-fat milk and a handful of blueberries
- Mid-Morning Snack: A handful of cashews and an orange
- Lunch: Tofu stir-fry with brown rice
- Afternoon Snack: Low-fat yogurt with flax seeds
- Dinner: Grilled chicken with sweet potato and roasted asparagus
- Evening Snack: An apple and a small handful of almonds

Day 3:

- Breakfast: Whole grain cereal with low-fat milk and a peach
- Mid-Morning Snack: A handful of walnuts and a banana
- Lunch: Baked fish with whole grain bread and a mixed vegetable salad
- Afternoon Snack: Low-fat yogurt with sunflower seeds
- Dinner: Tofu with quinoa and steamed green beans
- Evening Snack: A pear and a small handful of cashews

Day 4:

- Breakfast: Oatmeal with low-fat milk and a handful of strawberries
- Mid-Morning Snack: A handful of pecans and an apple
- Lunch: Grilled chicken wrap with whole grain tortilla
- Afternoon Snack: Low-fat yogurt with pumpkin seeds
- Dinner: Baked fish with sweet potato and roasted Brussels sprouts
- Evening Snack: An orange and a small handful of walnuts

Day 5:

- Breakfast: Whole grain cereal with low-fat milk and a handful of raspberries
- Mid-Morning Snack: A handful of almonds and a banana
- Lunch: Tofu salad with brown rice

- Afternoon Snack: Low-fat yogurt with chia seeds
- Dinner: Grilled chicken with quinoa and steamed carrots
- Evening Snack: A peach and a small handful of cashews

Day 6:

- Breakfast: Oatmeal with low-fat milk and a handful of blackberries
- Mid-Morning Snack: A handful of walnuts and an apple
- Lunch: Baked fish sandwich with whole grain bread
- Afternoon Snack: Low-fat yogurt with flax seeds
- Dinner: Tofu with sweet potato and roasted zucchini
- Evening Snack: An orange and a small handful of pecans

Day 7:

- Breakfast: Whole grain cereal with low-fat milk and a pear
- Mid-Morning Snack: A handful of cashews and a banana
- Lunch: Grilled chicken with brown rice and a mixed vegetable salad
- Afternoon Snack: Low-fat yogurt with sunflower seeds
- Dinner: Baked fish with quinoa and steamed spinach
- Evening Snack: An apple and a small handful of almonds

Also, don't forget to drink plenty of water throughout the day!

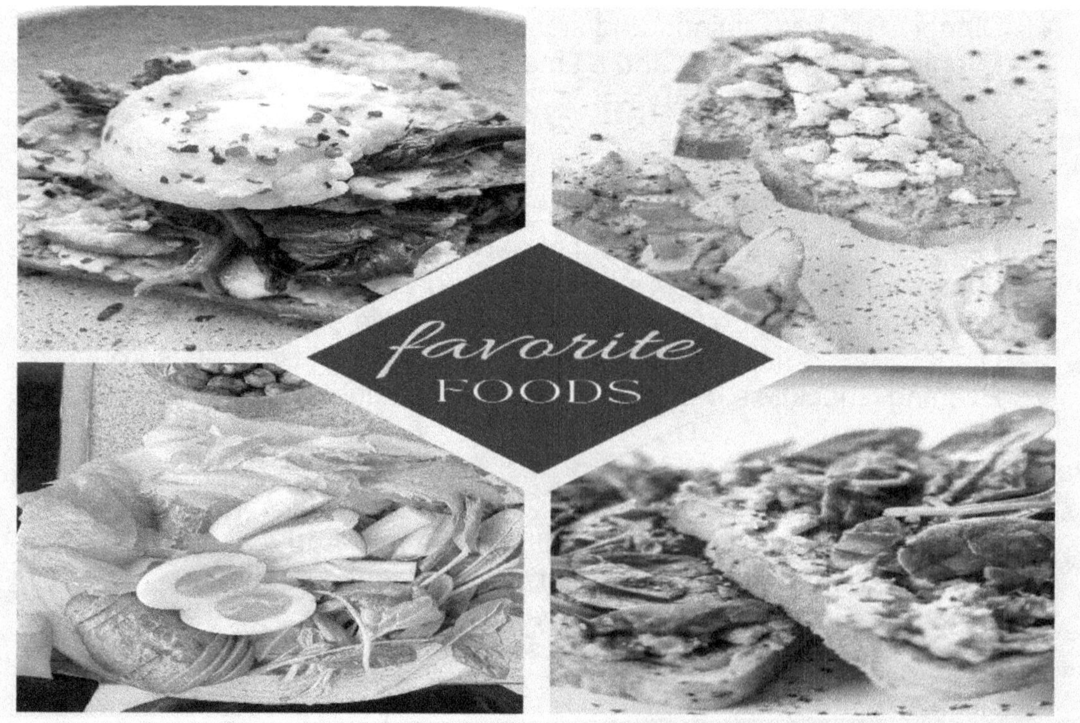

30 day healthy meal plan with a variety of different meals for each day:

Day 1:

Breakfast - Oatmeal with berries and almond milk

Lunch - Tuna salad sandwich on whole wheat bread, baby carrots, apple

Dinner - Chicken fajitas with peppers and onions, brown rice, salad

Day 2:

Breakfast - Greek yogurt with granola and blueberries

Lunch - Veggie and hummus wrap, mixed veggie salad

Dinner - Pasta primavera, garlic bread, caesar salad

Day 3:

Breakfast - Veggie omelet with whole wheat toast

Lunch - Lentil soup, whole grain crackers, grapes

Dinner - Salmon with dill sauce, quinoa pilaf, roasted brussels sprouts

Day 4:

Breakfast - Avocado toast with sliced tomatoes

Lunch - Grilled chicken Caesar salad

Dinner - Crispy baked fish tacos, pico de gallo, mexican rice

Day 5:

Breakfast - Protein smoothie with almond milk, banana, peanut butter

Lunch - Turkey burger with sweet potato fries

Dinner - Veggie and brown rice stir fry, miso soup

Day 6:

Breakfast - Overnight oats with chia seeds, almond milk, berries

Lunch - Spinach salad with hardboiled egg, feta cheese, balsamic dressing

Dinner - Beef and veggie kabobs, roasted potatoes, salad

Day 7:

Breakfast - Whole grain waffles topped with peanut butter and banana

Lunch - Veggie sandwich with hummus, tomato, avocado

Dinner - Chicken noodle soup, whole grain bread, mixed greens salad

Day 8:

Breakfast - Breakfast tacos with eggs, beans, salsa

Lunch - Quinoa tabbouleh salad

Dinner - Coconut curry shrimp, cauliflower rice

Day 9:

Breakfast - Peanut butter banana smoothie

Lunch - Grilled veggie and cheese sandwich

Dinner - Roasted pork tenderloin, sweet potatoes, green beans

Day 10:

Breakfast - Fruit and yogurt parfait with granola

Lunch - Chicken Caesar wrap with whole wheat tortilla

Dinner - Chili over baked potatoes, green salad

Day 11:

Breakfast - Veggie omelet with whole grain toast

Lunch - Tuna salad over mixed greens, apple

Dinner - Turkey meatballs, whole wheat pasta, roasted broccoli

Day 12:

Breakfast - Overnight oats with chia seeds, almond milk, and berries

Lunch - Falafel pita sandwich with veggies and hummus

Dinner - Teriyaki salmon, brown rice, stir fry veggies

Day 13:

Breakfast - Whole grain cereal with almond milk and banana

Lunch - Lentil vegetable soup, whole grain crackers

Dinner - Spaghetti squash bolognese, side salad

Day 14:

Breakfast - Veggie scramble with peppers, onions, spinach

Lunch - Greek salad with chicken, feta, pita bread

Dinner - Sheet pan fajitas with chicken, veggies, brown rice

Day 15:

Breakfast - Protein pancakes topped with peanut butter

Lunch - Grilled chicken sandwich, sweet potato fries

Dinner - Veggie fried rice with eggs, edamame

Day 16:

Breakfast - Yogurt parfait with granola and mixed berries

Lunch - Quinoa chickpea salad

Dinner - Pesto baked salmon, roasted asparagus

Day 17:

Breakfast - Breakfast burrito with eggs, cheese, salsa

Lunch - Chopped kale salad with chickpeas, feta, balsamic

Dinner - Chicken Parmesan over whole wheat linguine

Day 18:

Breakfast - Avocado toast with fried egg

Lunch - Vegetarian chili, corn bread

Dinner - Pork tenderloin, roasted veggies, baked potato

Day 19:

Breakfast - Overnight oats with peanut butter and bananas

Lunch - Tuna melt sandwich, carrot sticks

Dinner - Shrimp fajitas, sautéed peppers and onions, mexican rice

Day 20:

Breakfast - Veggie omelet with cheese, toast

Lunch - Chicken caesar salad

Dinner - Pasta with meatballs, side salad

Day 21:

Breakfast - Whole grain waffles with peanut butter

Lunch - Baked sweet potato stuffed with veggies and black beans

Dinner - Grilled salmon, quinoa pilaf, sauteed spinach

Day 22:

Breakfast - Greek yogurt with berries and granola

Lunch - Lentil and chickpea soup, whole grain roll

Dinner - Herb roasted chicken, potatoes, roasted carrots

Day 23:

Breakfast - Protein smoothie with banana, almond milk, peanut butter

Lunch - Veggie sandwich with hummus, avocado

Dinner - Zucchini noodle bolognese with turkey meat sauce

Day 24:

Breakfast - Breakfast tacos with scrambled eggs, salsa, cheese

Lunch - Quinoa tabbouleh salad

Dinner - Coconut curry chicken, cauliflower rice

Day 25:

Breakfast - Whole grain cereal with almond milk and blueberries

Lunch - Grilled chicken pita with veggies and hummus

Dinner - Baked cod with lemon, brown rice pilaf, green beans

Day 26:

Breakfast - Veggie egg scramble with toast

Lunch - Lentil soup, whole grain crackers

Dinner - Turkey chili over baked potato

Day 27:

Breakfast - Overnight oats with chia seeds, almond milk, banana

Lunch - Greek salad with salmon

Dinner - Veggie fried rice with tofu

Day 28:

Breakfast - Avocado toast with poached egg

Lunch - Falafel wrap with hummus and veggies

Dinner - Chicken fajitas with peppers and onions, brown rice

Day 29:

Breakfast - Breakfast sandwich with egg, cheese, whole wheat English muffin

Lunch - Chopped salad with chickpeas, chicken, balsamic dressing

Dinner - Pasta with marinara sauce, meatballs, side salad

Day 30:

Breakfast - Blueberry muffin, Greek yogurt, granola

Lunch - Grilled chicken sandwich, baked sweet potato fries

Dinner - Shrimp stir fry with veggies, brown rice

Also, don't forget to drink plenty of water throughout the day!

---

30 day meal plan with snacks scheduled after breakfast and lunch:

Day 1:

Breakfast - Oatmeal with berries and almond milk

Snack 1 - Hardboiled egg

Lunch - Tuna salad sandwich on whole wheat bread, baby carrots, apple

Snack 2 - Apple with peanut butter

Dinner - Chicken fajitas with peppers and onions, brown rice, salad

Day 2:

Breakfast - Greek yogurt with granola and blueberries

Snack 1 - Carrots and hummus

Lunch - Veggie and hummus wrap, mixed veggie salad

Snack 2 - Cottage cheese and berries

Dinner - Pasta primavera, garlic bread, caesar salad

Day 3:

Breakfast - Veggie omelet with whole wheat toast

Snack 1 - Celery with peanut butter

Lunch - Lentil soup, whole grain crackers, grapes

Snack 2 - Kale chips

Dinner - Salmon with dill sauce, quinoa pilaf, roasted brussels sprouts

Day 4:

Breakfast - Avocado toast with sliced tomatoes

Snack 1 - Whole grain crackers and cheese

Lunch - Grilled chicken caesar salad

Snack 2 - Trail mix

Dinner - Crispy baked fish tacos, pico de gallo, mexican rice

Day 5:

Breakfast - Protein smoothie with almond milk, banana, peanut butter

Snack 1 - Greek yogurt with berries

Lunch - Turkey burger with sweet potato fries

Snack 2 - Hummus and veggies

Dinner - Veggie and brown rice stir fry, miso soup

Day 6:

Breakfast - Overnight oats with chia seeds, almond milk, berries

Snack 1 - Apple with almond butter

Lunch - Spinach salad with hardboiled egg, feta cheese, balsamic dressing

Snack 2 - Roasted chickpeas

Dinner - Beef and veggie kabobs, roasted potatoes, salad

Day 7:

Breakfast - Whole grain waffles topped with peanut butter and banana

Snack 1 - Mixed nuts

Lunch - Veggie sandwich with hummus, tomato, avocado

Snack 2 - Protein shake

Dinner - Chicken noodle soup, whole grain bread, mixed greens salad

Day 8:

Breakfast - Breakfast tacos with eggs, beans, salsa

Snack 1 - Cottage cheese and pineapple

Lunch - Quinoa tabbouleh salad

Snack 2 - Celery sticks with nut butter

Dinner - Coconut curry shrimp, cauliflower rice

Day 9:

Breakfast - Peanut butter banana smoothie

Snack 1 - Whole grain crackers and cheese

Lunch - Grilled veggie and cheese sandwich

Snack 2 - Apple with sunflower seed butter

Dinner - Roasted pork tenderloin, sweet potatoes, green beans

Day 10:

Breakfast - Fruit and yogurt parfait with granola

Snack 1 - Trail mix

Lunch - Chicken caesar wrap with whole wheat tortilla

Snack 2 - Roasted chickpeas

Dinner - Chili over baked potatoes, green salad

Day 11:

Breakfast - Veggie omelet with whole grain toast

Snack 1 - Hardboiled egg

Lunch - Tuna salad over mixed greens, apple

Snack 2 - Banana with almond butter

Dinner - Turkey meatballs, whole wheat pasta, roasted broccoli

Day 12:

Breakfast - Overnight oats with chia seeds, almond milk, and berries

Snack 1 - Edamame

Lunch - Falafel pita sandwich with veggies and hummus

Snack 2 - Greek yogurt and berries

Dinner - Teriyaki salmon, brown rice, stir fry veggies

Day 13:

Breakfast - Whole grain cereal with almond milk and banana

Snack 1 - Carrots and hummus

Lunch - Lentil vegetable soup, whole grain crackers

Snack 2 - Cucumber slices with ranch dip

Dinner - Spaghetti squash bolognese, side salad

Day 14:

Breakfast - Veggie scramble with peppers, onions, spinach

Snack 1 - Cottage cheese and pineapples

Lunch - Greek salad with chicken, feta, pita bread

Snack 2 - Kale chips

Dinner - Sheet pan fajitas with chicken, veggies, brown rice

Day 15:

Breakfast - Protein pancakes topped with peanut butter

Snack 1 - Mixed nuts

Lunch - Grilled chicken sandwich, sweet potato fries

Snack 2 - Apple with sunflower seed butter

Dinner - Veggie fried rice with eggs, edamame

Day 16:

Breakfast - Yogurt parfait with granola and mixed berries

Snack 1 - Hummus and celery

Lunch - Quinoa chickpea salad

Snack 2 - Fresh berries

Dinner - Pesto baked salmon, roasted asparagus

Day 17:

Breakfast - Breakfast burrito with eggs, cheese, salsa

Snack 1 - Whole grain crackers and cheese

Lunch - Chopped kale salad with chickpeas, feta, balsamic

Snack 2 - Cucumber slices with hummus

Dinner - Chicken Parmesan over whole wheat linguine

Day 18:

Breakfast - Avocado toast with fried egg

Snack 1 - Protein shake

Lunch - Vegetarian chili, corn bread

Snack 2 - Carrots and ranch dip

Dinner - Pork tenderloin, roasted veggies, baked potato

Day 19:

Breakfast - Overnight oats with peanut butter and bananas

Snack 1 - Greek yogurt with granola

Lunch - Tuna melt sandwich, carrot sticks

Snack 2 - Celery with peanut butter

Dinner - Shrimp fajitas, sauteed peppers and onions, mexican rice

Day 20:

Breakfast - Veggie omelet with cheese, toast

Snack 1 - Apple slices with nut butter

Lunch - Chicken caesar salad

Snack 2 - Kale chips

Dinner - Pasta with meatballs, side salad

Day 21:

Breakfast - Whole grain waffles with peanut butter

Snack 1 - Hummus and veggies

Lunch - Baked sweet potato stuffed with veggies and black beans

Snack 2 - Cottage cheese and pineapple

Dinner - Grilled salmon, quinoa pilaf, sauteed spinach

Day 22:

Breakfast - Greek yogurt with berries and granola

Snack 1 - Hardboiled egg

Lunch - Lentil and chickpea soup, whole grain roll

Snack 2 - Mixed nuts

Dinner - Herb roasted chicken, potatoes, roasted carrots

Day 23:

Breakfast - Protein smoothie with banana, almond milk, peanut butter

Snack 1 - Apple with sunflower seed butter

Lunch - Veggie sandwich with hummus, avocado

Snack 2 - Carrots and hummus

Dinner - Zucchini noodle bolognese with turkey meat sauce

Day 24:

Breakfast - Breakfast tacos with scrambled eggs, salsa, cheese

Snack 1 - Cottage cheese and pineapple

Lunch - Quinoa tabbouleh salad

Snack 2 - Celery sticks with nut butter

Dinner - Coconut curry chicken, cauliflower rice

Day 25:

Breakfast - Whole grain cereal with almond milk and blueberries

Snack 1 - Greek yogurt with granola

Lunch - Grilled chicken pita with veggies and hummus

Snack 2 - Cucumber slices with ranch dip

Dinner - Baked cod with lemon, brown rice pilaf, green beans

Day 26:

Breakfast - Veggie egg scramble with toast

Snack 1 - Apple slices with peanut butter

Lunch - Lentil soup, whole grain crackers

Snack 2 - Kale chips

Dinner - Turkey chili over baked potato

Day 27:

Breakfast - Overnight oats with chia seeds, almond milk, banana

Snack 1 - Hummus and carrots

Lunch - Greek salad with salmon

Snack 2 - Hardboiled egg

Dinner - Veggie fried rice with tofu

Day 28:

Breakfast - Avocado toast with poached egg

Snack 1 - Mixed nuts

Lunch - Falafel wrap with hummus and veggies

Snack 2 - Fresh berries

Dinner - Chicken fajitas with peppers and onions, brown rice

Day 29:

Breakfast - Breakfast sandwich with egg, cheese, whole wheat English muffin

Snack 1 - Greek yogurt with granola

Lunch - Chopped salad with chickpeas, chicken, balsamic dressing

Snack 2 - Celery with peanut butter

Dinner - Pasta with marinara sauce, meatballs, side salad

Day 30:

Breakfast - Blueberry muffin, Greek yogurt, granola

Snack 1 - Apple with almond butter

Lunch - Grilled chicken sandwich, baked sweet potato fries

Snack 2 - Carrots and hummus

Dinner - Shrimp stir fry with veggies, brown rice

Also, don't forget to drink plenty of water throughout the day!

Another 30 day healthy meal plan with different variations:

Day 1:

Breakfast - Berry protein smoothie

Snack 1 - Hardboiled egg

Lunch - Grilled chicken salad with avocado, tomatoes

Snack 2 - Celery with almond butter

Dinner - Baked tilapia with veggies, brown rice

Day 2:

Breakfast - Spinach and feta omelet

Snack 1 - Cottage cheese and pineapple

Lunch - Turkey wrap with lettuce, tomato, hummus

Snack 2 - Apple slices with peanut butter

Dinner - Veggie and lentil soup, whole grain bread

Day 3:

Breakfast - Overnight oats with chia seeds, almond milk

Snack 1 - Carrots and hummus

Lunch - Tuna salad sandwich on whole wheat, lettuce, tomato

Snack 2 - Greek yogurt with mixed berries

Dinner - Veggie stir fry with tofu over quinoa

Day 4:

Breakfast - Avocado toast with egg

Snack 1 - Protein shake

Lunch - Chicken caesar salad

Snack 2 - Trail mix

Dinner - Salmon with sweet potato and roasted broccoli

Day 5:

Breakfast - Peanut butter and banana whole grain toast

Snack 1 - Cottage cheese and pineapple

Lunch - Falafel bowl with spinach, feta, hummus

Snack 2 - Apple with sunflower seed butter

Dinner - Turkey chili with beans over brown rice

Day 6:

Breakfast - Veggie scramble with peppers, onions, cheese

Snack 1 - Hardboiled egg

Lunch - Chicken pesto wrap with roasted veggies

Snack 2 - Kale chips

Dinner - Zucchini noodle Bolognese with turkey meatballs

Day 7:

Breakfast - Greek yogurt parfait with granola and berries

Snack 1 - Edamame

Lunch - Quinoa tabbouleh salad with chickpeas

Snack 2 - Cucumber slices with hummus

Dinner - Lemon garlic shrimp with roasted asparagus

Day 8:

Breakfast - Protein waffles with peanut butter

Snack 1 - Cottage cheese and pineapple

Lunch - Taco salad bowl with ground turkey

Snack 2 - Carrots and ranch dip

Dinner - Grilled chicken with baked potato and green beans

Day 9:

Breakfast - Breakfast tacos with eggs, beans, salsa

Snack 1 - Apple with almond butter

Lunch - Lentil and brown rice bowl

Snack 2 - Greek yogurt with granola

Dinner - Pesto pasta with grilled chicken and broccoli

Day 10:

Breakfast - Berry smoothie bowl with granola

Snack 1 - Roasted chickpeas

Lunch - Chopped kale salad with salmon

Snack 2 - Trail mix

Dinner - Pork tenderloin with roasted veggies

Day 11:

Breakfast - Veggie frittata

Snack 1 - Hummus and carrots

Lunch - Grilled chicken sandwich with avocado

Snack 2 - Mixed nuts

Dinner - Coconut curry chickpeas over cauliflower rice

Day 12:

Breakfast - Peanut butter overnight oats

Snack 1 - Hardboiled egg

Lunch - Beef and veggie kabobs with hummus

Snack 2 - Apple with almond butter

Dinner - Sheet pan fajitas with shrimp and veggies

Day 13:

Breakfast - Spinach and mushroom omelet

Snack 1 - Edamame

Lunch - Quinoa chickpea salad

Snack 2 - Kale chips

Dinner - Vegetarian chili over baked potato

Day 14:

Breakfast - Blueberry protein smoothie

Snack 1 - Carrots and hummus

Lunch - Mediterranean tuna salad over greens

Snack 2 - Cucumber slices with ranch

Dinner - Turkey meatloaf with roasted vegetables

Day 15:

Breakfast - Avocado toast with egg

Snack 1 - Greek yogurt with granola

Lunch - Grilled chicken pita with veggies

Snack 2 - Fresh berries

Dinner - Baked tilapia with brown rice and broccoli

Day 16:

Breakfast - Overnight oats with chia seeds

Snack 1 - Cottage cheese and pineapple

Lunch - Lentil and quinoa bowl

Snack 2 - Apple with sunflower seed butter

Dinner - Chicken Parmesan with whole wheat pasta

Day 17:

Breakfast - Spinach and goat cheese egg bake

Snack 1 - Mixed nuts

Lunch - Salmon burger with sweet potato fries

Snack 2 - Carrots and hummus

Dinner - Veggie stir fry with brown rice

Day 18:

Breakfast - Berry smoothie bowl

Snack 1 - Hardboiled egg

Lunch - Chicken caesar salad wrap

Snack 2 - Greek yogurt with granola

Dinner - Beef and broccoli stir fry with brown rice

Day 19:

Breakfast - Tofu veggie scramble

Snack 1 - Roasted chickpeas

Lunch - Falafel pita with hummus and veggies

Snack 2 - Apple with almond butter

Dinner - Fish tacos with cabbage slaw

Day 20:

Breakfast - Overnight oats with peanut butter

Snack 1 - Edamame

Lunch - Quinoa tabbouleh salad with tuna

Snack 2 - Trail mix

Dinner - Baked ziti with turkey sausage

Day 21:

Breakfast - Protein pancakes

Snack 1 - Cottage cheese and berries

Lunch - Chicken pesto sandwich

Snack 2 - Cucumber slices with hummus

Dinner - Lemon pepper cod with rice and spinach

Day 22:

Breakfast - Breakfast taco with scrambled egg

Snack 1 - Carrots and ranch dip

Lunch - Chopped chef salad with turkey

Snack 2 - Mixed nuts

Dinner - Veggie and chickpea curry with brown rice

Day 23:

Breakfast - Berry smoothie

Snack 1 - Hardboiled egg

Lunch - Grilled chicken pita with greens

Snack 2 - Apple with peanut butter

Dinner - Spaghetti squash bolognese

Day 24:

Breakfast - Veggie omelet

Snack 1 - Greek yogurt with granola

Lunch - Salmon salad over greens

Snack 2 - Kale chips

Dinner - Pork chops with roasted potatoes and carrots

Day 25:

Breakfast - Overnight oats with chia seeds

Snack 1 - Hummus and carrots

Lunch - Burrito bowl with rice, beans, chicken

Snack 2 - Fresh berries

Dinner - Pasta with meatballs and broccoli

Day 26:

Breakfast - Peanut butter toast with banana

Snack 1 - Cottage cheese and pineapple

Lunch - Chopped kale salad with chicken

Snack 2 - Apple with sunflower seed butter

Dinner - Fish tacos with cauliflower rice

Day 27:

Breakfast - Spinach and mushroom omelet

Snack 1 - Roasted chickpeas

Lunch - Lentil soup with whole grain bread

Snack 2 - Carrots and ranch dip

Dinner - Stuffed peppers with ground turkey

Day 28:

Breakfast - Acai bowl with granola

Snack 1 - Hardboiled egg

Lunch - Chicken pesto panini

Snack 2 - Cucumber slices with hummus

Dinner - Shrimp fried rice

Day 29:

Breakfast - Breakfast tacos with egg, cheese, salsa

Snack 1 - Mixed nuts

Lunch - Salmon salad with greens

Snack 2 - Greek yogurt with berries

Dinner - Tofu stir fry with veggies

Day 30:

Breakfast - Avocado toast with egg

Snack 1 - Edamame

Lunch - Quinoa and black bean bowl

Snack 2 - Apple with almond butter

Dinner - Veggie pizza with whole wheat crust

Also, don't forget to drink plenty of water throughout the day!

Recipes - Recipes for the 30 day meal plan:

Day 1 Breakfast - Oatmeal with Berries and Almond Milk:

- 1/2 cup rolled oats

- 1 cup almond milk

- 1/2 cup mixed berries

- 1 Tbsp. chopped almonds

- 1 tsp cinnamon

Cook oats in milk, top with berries and almonds.

Day 1 Lunch - Tuna Salad Sandwich:

- 1 can tuna, drained

- 2 Tbsp. mayo

- 1 stalk celery, diced

- 1 Tbsp. relish

- 1 tsp lemon juice

- 2 slices whole wheat bread

- Lettuce, tomato (optional)

Combine tuna, mayo, celery, relish and lemon juice. Serve on bread with veggies.

Day 1 Dinner - Chicken Fajitas:

- 1 lb. chicken breasts, sliced into strips

- 1 bell pepper, sliced

- 1 onion, sliced

- 2 tsp olive oil

- 1 tsp cumin

- 1 tsp chili powder

- 6 small whole wheat tortillas

- Toppings like salsa, cheese, etc.

Sauté chicken and veggies in oil and spices. Serve in tortillas with desired toppings.

Day 1 Snack 1

 - Hard Boiled Egg:

- Eggs

Place eggs in pot, cover with water. Bring to a boil, then simmer 12 min. Cool, peel and enjoy.

Day 1 Snack 2 - Apple with Peanut Butter:

- 1 apple, sliced

- 2 Tbsp. peanut butter

Slice apple and dip slices into peanut butter.

Day 2 Breakfast - Greek Yogurt with Granola and Blueberries:

- 1 cup Greek yogurt

- 1/4 cup granola

- 1/4 cup blueberries

Top yogurt with granola and blueberries.

Day 2 Lunch - Veggie and Hummus Wrap:

- 1 whole wheat tortilla

- 3-4 Tbsp. hummus

- Lettuce, tomato, cucumber, peppers

- 1/4 avocado, sliced

Spread hummus on tortilla, top with veggies and roll up.

Day 2 Dinner - Pasta Primavera:

- 8 oz. whole wheat pasta

- 1 cup mixed veggies (broccoli, carrots, peppers)

- 2 Tbsp. olive oil

- 2 cloves garlic, minced

- 1/4 cup pasta water

- Shredded parmesan cheese

Cook pasta according to package directions. In pan, sauté veggies in oil and garlic. Add pasta water to create sauce. Toss with pasta and parmesan.

Day 2 Snack 1 - Carrots and Hummus:

- Carrot sticks

- 2-3 Tbsp. hummus

Wash and cut carrots into sticks. Use for dipping hummus.

Day 2 Snack 2 - Cottage Cheese and Berries:

- 1/2 cup cottage cheese

- 1/2 cup mixed berries

Combine cottage cheese and berries in a bowl.

Day 3 Breakfast - Veggie Omelet:

- 2 eggs

- 1/4 cup diced peppers

- 1/4 cup diced onions

- 2 Tbsp. shredded cheese

- Salt and pepper

Whisk eggs, sauté veggies until soft. Add eggs, cook until set. Top with cheese.

Day 3 Lunch - Lentil Soup:

- 1 cup dried lentils

- 1 onion, diced

- 2 carrots, diced

- 4 cups broth

- 1 tsp cumin

- Salt and pepper

Simmer lentils and veggies in broth 20-30 min until soft. Season with cumin, salt and pepper.

Day 3 Snack 1 - Celery with Peanut Butter:

- Celery stalks

- 2 Tbsp. peanut butter

Spread peanut butter in celery stalks.

Day 3 Snack 2 - Kale Chips:

- Kale leaves

- 1 Tbsp. olive oil

- Seasonings like sea salt

Tear kale into pieces, toss with oil and seasonings. Bake at 375F for 5-10 min until crispy.

Day 3 Dinner - Salmon with Quinoa:

- 4 oz. salmon filet

- 1/2 cup quinoa

- 1 cup broth

- Lemon juice

- Roasted Brussels sprouts

Cook quinoa in broth. Bake salmon at 400F for 8-10 min. Roast brussels sprouts with olive oil. Squeeze lemon over salmon.

Day 4 Breakfast - Avocado Toast:

- 2 slices whole wheat bread

- 1/2 avocado, mashed

- 1 egg

- Everything bagel seasoning (optional)

Toast bread. Mash avocado on toast, top with fried egg. Sprinkle with seasoning if desired.

Day 4 Lunch - Grilled Chicken Caesar Salad:

- 4 oz. chicken breast, grilled

- 2 cups romaine lettuce, chopped

- 2 Tbsp. Caesar dressing

- 1/4 cup croutons

- Shredded parmesan cheese

Grill chicken breast. Toss lettuce with dressing, croutons and parmesan. Top with chicken.

Day 4 Dinner - Baked Fish Tacos:

- 4 oz. white fish like cod or tilapia

- 1 tsp chili powder

- 1 tsp cumin

- 2 corn tortillas

- Shredded cabbage, Pico de Gallo

Bake fish at 400F for 10-15 min with spices. Serve in tortillas with desired toppings.

Day 4 Snack 1 - Whole Grain Crackers and Cheese:

- 10 whole grain crackers

- 1 oz. cheddar cheese

Top crackers with sliced cheddar cheese.

Day 4 Snack 2 - Trail Mix:

- 1/4 cup nuts

- 1/4 cup dried fruit

- 1/4 cup seeds or granola

Combine nuts, seeds, granola and dried fruit in a bowl.

Day 5 Breakfast - Protein Smoothie:

- 1 scoop protein powder

- 1 banana

- 1 cup milk or yogurt

- 2 Tbsp. peanut butter

- Ice

Blend all ingredients until smooth.

Day 5 Lunch - Turkey Burger:

- 4 oz. ground turkey patty

- Whole wheat bun

- Lettuce, tomato, onion (toppings)

Grill patty. Serve on bun with veggies.

Day 5 Dinner - Brown Rice and Veggie Stir Fry:

- 1 cup brown rice

- 1 cup mixed veggies

- 2 Tbsp. soy sauce or teriyaki

- 1 Tbsp. oil

Cook rice. Heat oil, sauté veggies until tender. Add sauce and serve over rice.

Day 6 Breakfast - Overnight Oats:

- 1/2 cup oats

- 1/2 cup milk

- 2 Tbsp. chia seeds

- 1/2 cup berries

- 1 Tbsp. peanut butter

Combine oats, chia seeds, milk in a jar. Refrigerate overnight. Top with berries and peanut butter before eating.

Day 6 Lunch - Spinach Salad:

- 4 cups spinach

- 1 hardboiled egg, chopped

- 1/4 cup feta cheese

- 2 Tbsp. balsamic vinaigrette

Toss spinach with egg, feta and dressing.

Day 6 Dinner - Beef & Veggie Kabobs:

- 1 cup cubed beef

- 1 cup mixed veggies like onions, bell peppers, mushrooms

- 2 Tbsp. soy sauce

- 2 Tbsp. oil

Marinate beef and veggies in soy sauce and oil. Thread on skewers. Grill on high heat, turning occasionally until cooked through.

Day 6 Snack 1 - Apple with Almond Butter:

- 1 apple, sliced

- 2 Tbsp. almond butter

Spread almond butter on apple slices.

Day 6 Snack 2 - Roasted Chickpeas:

- 1 15-oz. can chickpeas, drained and rinsed

- 1 Tbsp. olive oil

- 1/2 tsp each salt, pepper, garlic powder

Toss chickpeas in oil and seasonings. Roast at 400F for 20 minutes, shaking halfway.

Day 7 Breakfast - Whole Grain Waffles:

- Make waffles from mix, or heat frozen whole grain waffles

- Top with peanut butter and sliced banana

Day 7 Lunch - Veggie Sandwich:

- 2 slices whole wheat bread

- 2-3 Tbsp. hummus

- Sliced veggies like tomato, cucumber, onion

- Lettuce

Spread hummus on bread. Layer toppings and enjoy.

Day 7 Dinner - Chicken Noodle Soup:

- 4 cups chicken broth

- 1 chicken breast, cooked and shredded

- 1 cup veggies like carrots, celery, onion

- 1 cup noodles

- Salt, pepper, seasoning to taste

Simmer veggies in broth. Add chicken, noodles and seasonings.

Day 7 Snack 1 - Mixed Nuts:

- 1/4 cup unsalted nuts like almonds, cashews, walnuts

Day 7 Snack 2 - Protein Shake:

- 1 scoop protein powder

- 1 cup milk or yogurt

- 1 banana

- Ice

Blend ingredients until smooth.

Day 8 Breakfast - Breakfast Tacos:

- 4 corn tortillas, warmed

- 4 eggs, scrambled

- 1/2 cup black beans

- Salsa

- Hot sauce (optional)

Scramble eggs with beans, season with salsa and hot sauce if desired. Serve in warm tortillas.

Day 8 Lunch - Quinoa Tabbouleh Salad:

- 1/2 cup dry quinoa, cooked

- 1 cup chopped parsley

- 1 cup chopped tomato

- 1/2 cup chopped cucumber

- 2 Tbsp. olive oil

- 2 Tbsp. lemon juice

- Salt and pepper to taste

Combine quinoa with veggies. Toss with oil, lemon juice and seasonings.

Day 8 Dinner - Coconut Curry Shrimp:

- 1 lb. shrimp, peeled and deveined

- 1 Tbsp. curry powder

- 1 (15 oz.) can coconut milk

- 1 cup veggies like onion, peppers, snap peas

- Serve over cauliflower rice

Sauté shrimp and veggies in coconut milk with curry powder. Serve over riced cauliflower.

Day 8 Snack 1 - Cottage Cheese with Pineapple:

- 1/2 cup cottage cheese

- 1/2 cup pineapple chunks

Day 8 Snack 2 - Celery with Nut Butter:

- Celery sticks

- 2 Tbsp. peanut or almond butter

Day 9 Breakfast - Peanut Butter Banana Smoothie:

- 1 banana

- 2 Tbsp. peanut butter

- 1 cup milk

- Ice

Blend all ingredients until smooth.

Day 9 Lunch - Grilled Cheese Sandwich:

- 2 slices whole wheat bread

- 2 slices cheddar cheese

- 2 Tbsp. butter

Butter outsides of bread. Grill sandwich over medium heat until bread is toasted and cheese melty.

Day 9 Dinner - Roasted Pork Tenderloin:

- 1 lb. pork tenderloin

- 2 Tbsp. olive oil

- Seasonings like garlic powder, paprika, salt

- Roasted sweet potatoes and green beans

Coat pork with oil and seasonings. Roast at 425F for 20 minutes until cooked through. Roast veggies tossed in oil.

Day 9 Snack 1 - Whole Grain Crackers with Cheese:

- 10 whole grain crackers

- 1 oz. sliced cheddar cheese

Day 9 Snack 2 - Apple with Sunflower Seed Butter:

- 1 apple, sliced

- 2 Tbsp. sunflower seed butter

Spread sunflower seed butter on apple slices.

Day 10 Breakfast - Yogurt Parfait:

- 1 cup Greek yogurt

- 1/2 cup mixed berries

- 1/4 cup granola

Layer ingredients in a bowl or jar.

Day 10 Lunch - Chicken Caesar Wrap:

- 1 whole wheat tortilla

- 3-4 oz. grilled chicken, sliced

- 2 Tbsp. Caesar dressing

- Shredded romaine lettuce

- Shredded parmesan cheese

Spread dressing on tortilla, layer with chicken, lettuce and cheese. Roll up tortilla.

Day 10 Dinner - Chili over Baked Potatoes:

- 1 lb. ground beef, cooked

- 1 15-oz can beans like kidney or black beans

- 1 14 oz. can diced tomatoes

- Chili powder, cumin, garlic to taste

- Baked potatoes, topped with chili

Cook beef with spices. Add tomatoes and beans. Serve over baked potatoes.

Day 10 Snack 1 - Trail Mix:

- 1/4 cup nuts

- 1/4 cup dried fruit like raisins, cranberries

- 1/4 cup granola or seeds

Mix ingredients together in a bowl.

Day 10 Snack 2 - Roasted Chickpeas:

- 1 15-oz. can chickpeas, drained and rinsed

- 1 Tbsp. olive oil

- 1/2 tsp each salt, pepper, garlic powder

Toss chickpeas in oil and seasonings. Roast at 400F for 20 minutes, shaking halfway.

Day 11 Breakfast - Veggie Omelet:

- 2 eggs, beaten

- 1/4 cup diced veggies like onion, pepper, spinach

- 2 Tbsp. shredded cheddar cheese

- Salt and pepper

Sauté veggies, pour in eggs. Cook until set, sprinkle cheese on top.

Day 11 Lunch - Tuna Salad:

- 1 can tuna, drained

- 1/4 cup plain Greek yogurt

- 1 Tbsp. lemon juice

- 1/4 cup diced celery

- Lettuce

Combine tuna, yogurt, lemon juice and celery. Serve on top of lettuce.

Day 11 Dinner - Turkey Meatballs:

- 1 lb. ground turkey

- 1/4 cup breadcrumbs

- 1 egg

- Seasonings like parsley, garlic powder

- Whole wheat pasta and roasted broccoli

Mix turkey, breadcrumbs, egg and seasonings. Form into balls, bake at 375F until cooked through. Serve with pasta and roasted broccoli.

Day 11 Snack 1 - Hard Boiled Egg- 1-2 eggs

Place eggs in a pot, cover with water. Bring to a boil, reduce to simmer for 12 minutes. Cool and peel.

Day 11 Snack 2 - Banana with Almond Butter:

- 1 banana, sliced

- 2 Tbsp. almond butter

Spread almond butter over banana slices.

Day 12 Breakfast - Overnight Oats:

- 1/2 cup oats

- 1/2 cup milk or yogurt

- 2 Tbsp. chia seeds

- 1/2 cup mixed berries

Combine oats, chia seeds and milk/yogurt in a jar or container. Refrigerate overnight. Top with berries before eating.

Day 12 Lunch - Falafel Pita:

- 4-5 baked or fried falafel patties

- 1 whole wheat pita

- Lettuce, tomato, cucumber, hummus

Stuff pita with falafel, veggies and hummus.

Day 12 Dinner - Teriyaki Salmon:

- 4-6 oz. salmon filet

- 2 Tbsp. teriyaki sauce

- 1 cup brown rice

- Stir fry veggies like broccoli, carrots, and onions

Marinate salmon in teriyaki sauce. Bake at 400F for 10 minutes until flaky. Serve over rice and veggies.

Day 12 Snack 1 - Edamame:

- 1/2 cup shelled edamame beans

Prepare according to package directions - boil in water or microwave.

Day 12 Snack 2 - Greek Yogurt with Berries:

- 1 cup plain Greek yogurt

- 1/2 cup mixed berries

Day 13 Breakfast - Whole Grain Cereal:

- 1 cup whole grain cereal like bran flakes or shredded wheat

- 1 cup milk or yogurt

- Sliced banana

Add milk and top with sliced banana.

Day 13 Lunch - Lentil Vegetable Soup:

- 1 cup dried lentils

- 4 cups vegetable broth

- 1 onion, diced

- 2 carrots, diced

- 2 stalks celery, diced

- 1 bay leaf

- Salt and pepper to taste

Simmer lentils and veggies in broth for 30 minutes until soft. Season with salt and pepper.

Day 13 Dinner - Spaghetti Squash Bolognese:

- 1 spaghetti squash, roasted into noodles

- 1/2 lb. Ground turkey

- 1/2 onion, diced

- 1/2 cup marinara sauce

- Parmesan cheese

Sauté turkey and onion, add marinara. Toss with spaghetti squash noodles. Top with parmesan.

Day 13 Snack 1 - Carrots and Hummus:

- Carrot sticks, washed

- 2-3 Tbsp. hummus

Day 13 Snack 2 - Cucumber Slices with Ranch:

- Cucumber, sliced

- 2 Tbsp. ranch dressing

Use ranch for dipping cucumber slices.

Day 14 Breakfast - Veggie Scramble:

- 2 eggs, beaten

- 1/4 cup diced peppers and onions

- Handful baby spinach

- 2 Tbsp. shredded cheddar cheese

Sauté veggies, pour in eggs. Cook until set, top with cheese.

Day 14 Lunch - Greek Salad:

- 2 cups chopped romaine lettuce

- 1/4 cup chickpeas

- 1/4 cup diced cucumbers

- 1/4 cup crumbled feta cheese

- 2 Tbsp. Greek dressing

- 4 oz. grilled chicken breast, sliced

- Whole wheat pita wedges

Toss salad ingredients together. Top with chicken and serve with pita wedges.

Day 14 Dinner - Sheet Pan Fajitas:

- 1 lb. Chicken breasts, sliced into strips

- 1 red bell pepper, sliced

- 1 onion, sliced

- 2 tsp chili powder

- 1 tsp. cumin

- Pinch cayenne pepper

- Lime wedges

Toss chicken and veggies with spices. Roast at 425F 15-20 minutes. Serve with lime.

Day 14 Snack 1 - Cottage Cheese with Pineapple:

- 1/2 cup cottage cheese

- 1/2 cup pineapple chunks

Day 14 Snack 2 - Kale Chips:

- 4 cups kale leaves, torn into pieces

- 1 Tbsp. olive oil

- Sea salt

Toss kale with oil and salt. Bake at 375F for 5 minutes until crispy.

Day 15 Breakfast - Protein Pancakes:

- Make from protein powder pancake mix, or use favorite whole grain recipe

- Top with 2 Tbsp. peanut butter

Day 15 Lunch - Grilled Chicken Sandwich:

- 4 oz. Chicken breast, grilled

- 2 slices whole wheat bread

- Lettuce, tomato, onion (optional toppings)

- 2 tsp mustard or mayo if desired

Assemble sandwich with chicken and toppings.

Day 15 Dinner - Veggie Fried Rice:

- 1 cup brown rice, cooked

- 1 cup mixed diced veggies like carrot, onion, bell pepper

- 2 eggs, scrambled

- 2 Tbsp. Soy sauce

- 1 tsp. sesame oil

Stir fry rice, veggies and eggs. Toss with soy sauce and sesame oil.

Day 15 Snack 1 - Mixed Nuts:

- 1/4 cup unsalted nuts like almonds, cashews, pecans

Day 15 Snack 2 - Apple with Sunflower Seed Butter:

- 1 apple, sliced

- 2 Tbsp. sunflower seed butter

Spread seed butter over apple slices.

Day 16 Breakfast - Yogurt Parfait:

- 1 cup Greek yogurt

- 1/2 cup mixed berries

- 2 Tbsp. granola

Layer ingredients in a bowl or jar.

Day 16 Lunch - Quinoa Chickpea Salad:

- 1/2 cup quinoa, cooked

- 1/2 cup chickpeas, rinsed and drained

- 1/4 cup chopped cucumber

- 1/4 cup diced tomato

- 2 Tbsp. lemon juice

- 2 Tbsp. olive oil

- Salt and pepper to taste

Combine quinoa, chickpeas and veggies. Toss with lemon juice, oil and seasonings.

Day 16 Dinner - Pesto Salmon:

- 4 oz. salmon filet

- 2 Tbsp. pesto

- Roasted asparagus

Spread pesto over salmon. Bake at 400F for 10 minutes until flaky. Roast asparagus tossed in olive oil.

Day 16 Snack 1 - Hummus and Celery:

- 2-3 Tbsp. hummus

- Celery sticks

Day 16 Snack 2 - Berries:

- 1 cup mixed berries like blueberries, raspberries, blackberries

Day 17 Breakfast - Breakfast Burrito:

- 1 whole wheat tortilla

- 2 scrambled eggs

- 2 Tbsp. shredded cheddar cheese

- 2 Tbsp. salsa

Warm tortilla. Add scrambled egg, cheese and salsa, wrap up burrito style.

Day 17 Lunch - Kale Salad:

- 4 cups chopped kale

- 1/4 cup chickpeas

- 1/4 cup feta cheese

- 2 Tbsp. balsamic vinaigrette

Massage kale with dressing. Top with chickpeas and feta.

Day 17 Dinner - Chicken Parmesan:

- 4 oz. chicken breast

- 2 Tbsp. marinara sauce

- 2 Tbsp. parmesan cheese

- Whole wheat linguine

- Steamed broccoli

Bread chicken breast, cook until done. Top with sauce and cheese. Serve with pasta and broccoli.

Day 17 Snack 1 - Whole Grain Crackers and Cheese:

- 10 whole grain crackers

- 1 oz. cheddar cheese, sliced

Day 17 Snack 2 - Cucumber and Hummus:

- Cucumber slices

- 2-3 Tbsp. hummus

Day 18 Breakfast - Avocado Toast:

- 2 slices whole wheat toast

- 1/2 mashed avocado

- 1 fried egg

- Everything bagel seasoning (optional)

Toast bread, mash avocado on top. Add fried egg and sprinkle with seasoning if desired.

Day 18 Lunch - Vegetarian Chili:

- 1 15-oz can beans like kidney, chickpeas or black beans

- 14 oz. can diced tomatoes

- 1 cup veggies like onion, bell pepper, carrots

- Chili powder, cumin, garlic to taste

- Serve over corn bread

Simmer all ingredients until thickened, about 20 minutes.

Day 18 Dinner - Pork Tenderloin:

- 4 oz. pork tenderloin

- 2 tsp olive oil

- 1/4 tsp each salt and pepper

- Roasted potatoes and veggies

Rub pork with oil and seasonings. Roast at 425F for 15-20 minutes until cooked through. Roast potatoes and veggies tossed in oil.

Day 18 Snack 1 - Protein Shake:

- 1 scoop protein powder

- 1 banana

- 1 cup milk or yogurt

- Ice

Blend all ingredients until smooth and creamy.

Day 18 Snack 2 - Carrots and Ranch Dip:

- Carrot sticks

- 2 Tbsp. ranch dressing

Day 19 Breakfast - Overnight Oats:

- 1/2 cup oats

- 1/2 cup milk or yogurt

- 1 Tbsp. peanut butter

- 1/2 banana, sliced

- Cinnamon

Combine oats, milk, and peanut butter in jar. Refrigerate overnight. Top with banana before eating.

Day 19 Lunch - Tuna Melt:

- 1 can tuna, drained

- 1/4 cup plain Greek yogurt

- 1 tsp lemon juice

- 2 slices whole wheat bread

- 2 slices cheddar cheese

- Tomato slices

Mix tuna, yogurt and lemon juice. Toast bread, top tuna mix and cheese. Broil until melted.

Day 19 Dinner - Shrimp Fajitas:

- 12 large shrimp, peeled

- 1 red bell pepper, sliced

- 1/2 onion, sliced

- 2 tsp olive oil

- 1 tsp chili powder

- 1 tsp cumin

- 6 small whole wheat tortillas

Sauté shrimp and veggies in oil and spices. Wrap in tortillas with toppings like salsa or guacamole.

Day 19 Snack 1 - Greek Yogurt with Granola:

- 1 cup Greek yogurt

- 1/4 cup granola

Day 19 Snack 2 - Celery with Peanut Butter:

- Celery sticks

- 1-2 Tbsp. peanut butter

Day 20 Breakfast - Veggie Omelet:

- 2 eggs, beaten

- 1/4 cup diced onion, pepper, mushrooms

- 2 Tbsp. shredded cheese

- Salt and pepper

Sauté veggies, pour in eggs to cook until set. Top with cheese.

Day 20 Lunch - Chicken Caesar Salad:

- 4 oz. grilled chicken, sliced

- 2 cups chopped romaine

- 2 Tbsp. Caesar dressing

- 1/4 cup croutons

- Shredded parmesan (optional)

Toss romaine with dressing, croutons and parmesan. Top with chicken.

Day 20 Dinner - Pasta with Meatballs:

- 4-5 frozen or homemade meatballs

- 8 oz. whole wheat pasta

- 1/2 cup marinara sauce

- Steamed broccoli

Day 20 Snack 1 - Apple Slices with Nut Butter:

- 1 apple, sliced

- 1-2 Tbsp. peanut or almond butter

Day 20 Snack 2 - Kale Chips:

- 4 cups kale leaves, torn into pieces

- 1 Tbsp. olive oil

- Sea salt

Toss kale with oil and salt. Bake at 375F for 5 minutes until crispy.

Day 21 Breakfast - Whole Grain Waffles with Peanut Butter:

- Make waffles from mix or heat frozen whole grain waffles

- Top with 2 Tbsp. peanut butter

Day 21 Lunch - Baked Sweet Potato:

- 1 medium sweet potato

- 1/4 cup black beans

- 1/4 cup salsa

- 2 Tbsp. shredded cheese

Poke holes in potato, bake at 425F 45 minutes until tender. Split open, top with beans, salsa and cheese.

Day 21 Dinner - Grilled Salmon:

- 4 oz. salmon fillet

- Lemon wedges

- 1/2 cup quinoa

- 1 cup steamed spinach

Grill salmon 5 minutes per side. Squeeze lemon juice over top. Serve with quinoa and spinach.

Day 21 Snack 1 - Hummus and Veggies:

- Carrot sticks, bell pepper strips

- 2-3 Tbsp. hummus

Day 21 Snack 2 - Cottage Cheese with Pineapple:

- 1/2 cup cottage cheese

- 1/2 cup pineapple chunks

Day 22 Breakfast - Greek Yogurt with Berries and Granola:

- 1 cup Greek yogurt

- 1/2 cup mixed berries

- 2 Tbsp. granola

Day 22 Lunch - Lentil and Chickpea Soup:

- 1/2 cup dried lentils

- 1/2 cup chickpeas

- 1 onion, diced

- 4 cups vegetable broth

- 1 bay leaf

- Salt and pepper to taste

Simmer lentils, chickpeas and onion in broth for 30 minutes until soft. Season with salt and pepper.

Day 22 Dinner - Herb Roasted Chicken:

- 4 oz. chicken breast

- 1 tsp olive oil

- 1/4 tsp each basil, oregano, thyme

- Roasted potatoes and carrots

Coat chicken with oil and herbs. Roast at 400F for 15-20 minutes until cooked through. Toss potatoes and carrots in oil, roast.

Day 22 Snack 1 - Hard Boiled Egg:

- 1 egg

Place in boiling water for 12 minutes. Cool, peel and enjoy.

Day 22 Snack 2 - Mixed Nuts:

- 1/4 cup unsalted nuts like almonds, cashews, walnuts

Day 23 Breakfast - Banana Peanut Butter Protein Smoothie:

- 1 banana

- 1 scoop protein powder

- 1 cup milk

- 2 Tbsp. peanut butter

- Ice

Blend all ingredients until smooth.

Day 23 Lunch - Veggie Sandwich with Hummus:

- 2 slices whole wheat bread

- 3-4 Tbsp. hummus

- Lettuce, tomato, cucumber, bell pepper

Spread hummus on bread. Layer with veggies.

Day 23 Dinner - Zucchini Noodle Bolognese:

- 2 medium zucchini, spiralized

- 1/2 lb. Ground turkey

- 1/2 onion, diced

- 1/2 cup marinara sauce

Sauté turkey and onion, add sauce. Toss with zucchini noodles.

Day 23 Snack 1 - Apple with Sunflower Seed Butter:

- 1 apple, sliced

- 2 Tbsp. sunflower seed butter

Day 23 Snack 2 - Carrots with Hummus:

- Carrot sticks

- 2-3 Tbsp. hummus

Day 24 Breakfast - Breakfast Tacos:

- 3 corn tortillas, warmed

- 3 eggs, scrambled

- 2 Tbsp. shredded cheddar cheese

- Salsa

Fill tortillas with scrambled eggs, cheese and salsa.

Day 24 Lunch - Quinoa Tabbouleh:

- 1/2 cup quinoa, cooked

- 1/2 cup diced tomato

- 1/2 cup diced cucumber

- 1/4 cup chopped parsley

- 2 Tbsp. olive oil

- 2 Tbsp. lemon juice

Combine quinoa with veggies. Toss with oil and lemon juice.

Day 24 Dinner - Coconut Curry Chicken:

- 4 oz. chicken, diced

- 1/2 cup light coconut milk

- 1 Tbsp. red curry paste

- 1 cup veggies like onion, peppers, snap peas

- Cauliflower rice

Simmer chicken and veggies in coconut milk with curry paste. Serve over riced cauliflower.

Day 24 Snack 1 - Cottage Cheese with Pineapple:

- 1/2 cup cottage cheese

- 1/2 cup pineapple chunks

Day 24 Snack 2 - Celery with Nut Butter:

- Celery sticks

- 1-2 Tbsp. almond or peanut butter

Day 25 Breakfast - Whole Grain Cereal:

- 1 cup whole grain cereal like bran flakes or shredded wheat

- 1 cup milk or yogurt

- 1/2 cup blueberries

Day 25 Lunch - Chicken Pita:

- 1 whole wheat pita

- 3-4 oz. grilled chicken, sliced

- Lettuce, tomato, cucumber, hummus

Stuff pita with chicken, veggies and hummus.

Day 25 Dinner - Baked Cod:

- 4 oz. cod fillet

- Lemon wedges

- 1/2 cup brown rice pilaf

- 1 cup green beans

Bake cod at 400F for 10-12 minutes until flaky. Squeeze lemon over top. Serve with rice pilaf and green beans.

Day 25 Snack 1 - Greek Yogurt with Granola:

- 1 cup Greek yogurt

- 2 Tbsp. granola

Day 25 Snack 2 - Cucumber Slices with Ranch:

- Cucumber, sliced

- 2 Tbsp. ranch dressing

Day 26 Breakfast - Veggie Egg Scramble:

- 2 eggs, beaten

- 1/4 cup diced onion, pepper, tomato

- 2 Tbsp. shredded cheddar cheese

Sauté veggies, pour in eggs. Cook until set, top with cheese.

Day 26 Lunch - Lentil Soup:

- 1/2 cup dried lentils

- 1 onion, diced

- 2 carrots, diced

- 4 cups vegetable broth

- 1 bay leaf

- Salt and pepper to taste

Simmer lentils and veggies in broth until soft, about 30 minutes. Season with salt and pepper.

Day 26 Dinner - Turkey Chill over Baked Potato:

- 4 oz. ground turkey, browned

- 14 oz. can diced tomatoes

- 15 oz. can kidney beans, drained

- Chili powder, cumin, garlic to taste

- Top baked potato

Cook turkey in spices, add tomatoes and beans. Simmer 15 minutes. Serve over baked potato.

Day 26 Snack 1 - Apple Slices with Peanut Butter:

- 1 apple, sliced

- 1-2 Tbsp. peanut butter

Day 26 Snack 2 - Kale Chips:

- 4 cups torn kale leaves

- 1 Tbsp. olive oil

- Sea salt

Massage kale with oil and salt. Bake at 375F for 5 minutes until crispy.

Day 27 Breakfast - Overnight Oats:

- 1/2 cup rolled oats

- 1/2 cup milk or yogurt

- 1 Tbsp. chia seeds

- 1/2 banana, mashed

Combine oats, chia seeds, milk and banana in jar. Refrigerate overnight.

Day 27 Lunch - Greek Salad with Salmon:

- 2 cups chopped romaine lettuce

- 1/4 cup chickpeas

- 1/4 cup diced cucumber

- 1/4 cup crumbled feta

- 4 oz. salmon, grilled or baked

Toss salad ingredients, top with salmon.

Day 27 Dinner - Tofu Veggie Fried Rice:

- 1 cup brown rice, cooked

- 1 cup mixed diced veggies

- 8 oz. firm tofu, cubed

- 2 eggs, scrambled

- 2 Tbsp. soy sauce

Stir fry rice, tofu, eggs and veggies. Toss with soy sauce.

Day 27 Snack 1 - Hummus and Carrots:

- About 5 carrot sticks

- 2-3 Tbsp. hummus

Day 27 Snack 2 - Hard Boiled Egg:

- 1 egg

Place in boiling water for 12 minutes. Cool, peel and enjoy.

Day 28 Breakfast - Avocado Toast:

- 2 slices whole wheat toast

- 1/2 avocado, mashed

- 1 fried egg

- Red pepper flakes (optional)

Toast bread. Mash avocado on top, add egg. Sprinkle with red pepper flakes if desired.

Day 28 Lunch - Falafel Wrap:

- 4-5 baked or fried falafel pattles, crumbled

- 1 whole wheat tortilla

- Lettuce, tomato, cucumber, hummus

Fill tortilla with falafel, veggies and hummus. Roll up.

Day 28 Dinner - Chicken Fajitas:

- 4 oz. chicken breast, sliced

- 1/2 bell pepper, sliced

- 1/2 onion, sliced

- 1 tsp chili powder

- 1 tsp cumin

- 3 small whole wheat tortillas

- Toppings like salsa, guacamole

Sauté chicken and veggies in spices. Serve in tortillas with desired toppings.

Day 28 Snack 1 - Mixed Nuts:

- 1/4 cup nuts like almonds, cashews, walnuts

Day 28 Snack 2 - Berries:

- About 1 cup mixed berries

Day 29 Breakfast - Breakfast Sandwich:

- 1 whole wheat English muffin

- 1 egg, fried or scrambled

- 1 slice cheddar cheese

- 1 slice tomato (optional)

Toast muffin, top with egg, cheese and tomato if desired.

Day 29 Lunch - Chicken Chopped Salad:

- 2 cups chopped romaine

- 1/4 cup chickpeas

- 4 oz. grilled chicken, chopped

- 1 Tbsp. balsamic vinaigrette

Toss salad ingredients and dressing together.

Day 29 Dinner - Whole Wheat Pasta with Meatballs:

- 8 oz. whole wheat pasta

- 4-5 frozen or homemade meatballs, cooked

- 1/2 cup marinara sauce

- Steamed broccoli

Cook pasta according to package directions. Add sauce, meatballs and vegetables.

Day 29 Snack 1 - Greek Yogurt with Granola:

- 1 cup Greek yogurt

- 2 Tbsp. granola

Day 29 Snack 2 - Celery with Peanut Butter:

- 3-4 celery sticks

- 1-2 Tbsp. peanut butter

Day 30 Breakfast - Blueberry Muffin:

- 1 whole wheat blueberry muffin

- 1 cup Greek yogurt

- 1/4 cup granola

Day 30 Lunch - Grilled Chicken Sandwich:

- 1 whole wheat bun

- 4 oz. grilled chicken breast

- Lettuce, tomato, onion (optional toppings)

- 1 tsp mustard or mayo (optional)

Day 30 Dinner - Shrimp Stir Fry:

- 8-10 shrimp, peeled and deveined

- 1 cup mixed stir fry veggies

- 1 Tbsp. olive oil

- 1 Tbsp. soy sauce

- 1 cup brown rice

Sauté shrimp and vegetables in oil. Toss with soy sauce. Serve over brown rice.

Day 30 Snack 1 - Apple with Almond Butter:

- 1 apple, sliced

- 1-2 Tbsp. almond butter

Day 30 Snack 2 - Carrots with Hummus:

- About 5 carrot sticks

- 2-3 Tbsp. hummus

Also, don't forget to drink plenty of water throughout the day!

---

30 day healthy meal plan with additional details for each meal and snack:

Day 1

Breakfast - Oatmeal with Berries and Almond Milk

- 1/2 cup oats (150 calories, 5g protein, 27g carbs, 3g fat)

- 1 cup unsweetened almond milk (30 calories, 1g protein, 1g carb, 2.5g fat)

- 1/2 cup mixed berries (blackberries, raspberries, blueberries) (40 calories, 1g protein, 10g carbs, 0.5g fat)

- 1 Tbsp. Slivered almonds (35 calories, 2g protein, 3g carbs, 3g fat)

- 1 tsp cinnamon

- Directions: Combine oats and milk in a microwave-safe bowl. Microwave for 2-3 minutes until thickened. Top with berries and almonds. Sprinkle cinnamon on top.

Snack 1 - Hard Boiled Egg

- 1 large egg (80 calories, 6g protein, 0g carbs, 6g fat)

- Directions: Place egg in a small pot and cover with water. Bring to a boil then reduce to simmer for 12 minutes. Cool under running water and peel.

Lunch - Tuna Salad Sandwich

- 3 oz. canned tuna in water (90 calories, 21g protein, 0g carbs, 1g fat)

- 2 Tbsp. Light mayo (60 calories, 0g protein, 0g carbs, 7g fat)

- 1 stalk celery, diced (5 calories, 0g protein, 1g carb, 0g fat)

- 1 Tbsp. Sweet pickle relish (15 calories, 0g protein, 4g carbs, 0g fat)

- 1 tsp lemon juice (1 calorie, 0g protein, 0g carbs, 0g fat)

- 2 slices whole wheat bread (140 calories, 8g protein, 24g carbs, 2g fat)

- Lettuce, tomato, onion (optional)

- Directions: In a bowl, mix tuna, mayo, celery relish and lemon juice. Toast bread if desired. Assemble sandwich with tuna salad and vegetable toppings.

Snack 2 - Apple with Peanut Butter

- 1 small apple, sliced (80 calories, 0g protein, 21g carbs, 0g fat)

- 2 Tbsp. Natural peanut butter (190 calories, 8g protein, 6g carbs, 16g fat)

- Directions: Spread peanut butter over apple slices.

Dinner - Chicken Fajitas

- 4 oz. boneless, skinless chicken breast, sliced (120 calories, 26g protein, 0g carbs, 1.5g fat)

- 1/2 red bell pepper, sliced (20 calories, 1g protein, 5g carbs, 0g fat)

- 1/2 onion, sliced (30 calories, 1g protein, 7g carbs, 0g fat)

- 1 tsp olive oil (40 calories, 0g protein, 0g carbs, 4g fat)

- 1/2 tsp cumin

- 1/2 tsp chili powder

- 2 small (6-inch) whole wheat tortillas (100 calories, 4g protein, 18g carbs, 1g fat each)

- Optional toppings like salsa, light sour cream, shredded lettuce

- Directions: Heat oil in skillet over medium-high heat. Add chicken and cook 5-6 minutes until no longer pink inside. Add bell pepper, onion and spices; cook 2-3 more minutes until softened. Serve chicken and veggie mixture over tortillas with desired toppings.

Day 1 Totals: Calories - 1260, Protein - 92g, Carbs - 178g, Fat - 48g

Day 2

Breakfast - Greek Yogurt with Granola and Blueberries

- 1 cup nonfat plain Greek yogurt (100 calories, 18g protein, 9g carbs, 0g fat)

- 1/4 cup low-fat granola (110 calories, 3g protein, 18g carbs, 2g fat)

- 1/4 cup blueberries (20 calories, 0g protein, 5g carbs, 0g fat)

- Directions: In a bowl or container, layer yogurt, granola and blueberries. Enjoy immediately or refrigerate overnight.

Snack 1 - Carrots with Hummus

- 5-6 medium carrots, cleaned and cut into sticks (50 calories, 1g protein, 12g carbs, 0g fat)

- 2 Tbsp. hummus (50 calories, 2g protein, 4g carbs, 3g fat)

- Directions: Arrange carrot sticks on plate or in container. Use hummus as a dip.

Lunch - Veggie and Hummus Wrap

- 1 whole wheat tortilla (100 calories, 4g protein, 18g carbs, 1g fat)

- 3 Tbsp. hummus (75 calories, 3g protein, 6g carbs, 5g fat)

- Fillings: lettuce, tomato, cucumber slices, bell pepper strips (30 calories, 2g protein, 6g carbs, 0g fat)

- 1/4 avocado, sliced (60 calories, 1g protein, 3g carbs, 6g fat)

- Directions: Spread hummus evenly over tortilla. Layer vegetable fillings and sliced avocado. Roll up tightly.

Snack 2 - Cottage Cheese with Berries

- 1/2 cup low-fat cottage cheese (80 calories, 14g protein, 3g carbs, 1g fat)

- 1/2 cup mixed berries (strawberries, blueberries, raspberries) (40 calories, 1g protein, 10g carbs, 0.5g fat)

- Directions: Spoon cottage cheese into bowl or container. Top with mixed berries.

Dinner - Pasta Primavera

- 2 oz. dry whole wheat pasta (200 calories, 8g protein, 40g carbs, 1.5g fat)

- 1 cup mixed vegetables (broccoli, carrots, bell peppers), chopped (30 calories, 2g protein, 7g carbs, 0g fat)

- 1 tsp olive oil (40 calories, 0g protein, 0g carbs, 4g fat)

- 2 cloves garlic, minced

- 2 Tbsp. Shredded parmesan cheese (20 calories, 2g protein, 0g carbs, 1g fat)

- Directions: Cook pasta according to package directions. In a skillet, cook vegetables in oil and garlic until tender. Toss with pasta and cheese.

Day 2 Totals: Calories - 1295, Protein - 77g, Carbs - 167g, Fat - 30g

Day 3

Breakfast - Veggie Omelet with Whole Wheat Toast

- 2 eggs (140 calories, 12g protein, 0g carbs, 10g fat)

- 1/4 cup diced bell pepper (10 calories, 0g protein, 2g carbs, 0g fat)

- 1/4 cup diced onion (15 calories, 0g protein, 4g carbs, 0g fat)

- 2 Tbsp. Shredded cheddar cheese (50 calories, 4g protein, 0g carbs, 4g fat)

- Salt and pepper to taste

- 1 slice whole wheat toast (70 calories, 4g protein, 12g carbs, 1g fat)

- Directions: Whisk eggs in a bowl with a fork. Heat a small nonstick skillet over medium heat and coat with cooking spray. Add peppers and onion and cook for 3-5 minutes until softened. Pour in eggs. As eggs start to cook, gently move eggs around pan with a spatula. Cook until set then sprinkle cheese on top. Season with salt and pepper. Serve omelet with whole wheat toast.

Snack 1 - Celery with Peanut Butter

- 4 celery sticks (5 calories, 0g protein, 1g carb, 0g fat)

- 1 Tbsp. Natural peanut butter (95 calories, 4g protein, 3g carbs, 8g fat)

- Directions: Clean and cut celery if needed. Use celery sticks to scoop up peanut butter for dipping.

Lunch - Lentil Soup

- 1/2 cup dried lentils (230 calories, 17g protein, 40g carbs, 1g fat)

- 1 small onion, diced (40 calories, 1g protein, 9g carbs, 0g fat)

- 2 medium carrots, diced (35 calories, 1g protein, 8g carbs, 0g fat)

- 4 cups low-sodium vegetable broth (20 calories, 2g protein, 2g carbs, 0g fat)

- 1 tsp cumin

- Salt and pepper to taste

- 5 whole grain crackers (25 calories, 1g protein, 5g carbs, 0g fat per cracker)

- 1/2 cup red grapes (52 calories, 0g protein, 13g carbs, 0.3g fat)

- Directions: Rinse lentils and dice veggies. In a pot, combine lentils, onion, carrots, broth and cumin. Bring to a boil, then reduce to a simmer for 20-30 minutes, until lentils are tender. Season with salt and pepper. Serve with whole grain crackers and grapes on the side.

Snack 2 - Kale Chips

- 2 cups torn kale leaves (20 calories, 2g protein, 4g carbs, 0g fat)

- 1 tsp olive oil (40 calories, 0g protein, 0g carbs, 4g fat)

- Sea salt to taste

- Directions: Tear kale leaves into bite size pieces discarding thick stems. Toss with oil and season with sea salt. Arrange in a single layer on a baking sheet. Bake at 375°F for 5 minutes, until crisp but not burnt.

Dinner - Baked Salmon

- 4 oz. salmon fillet (180 calories, 22g protein, 0g carbs, 10g fat)

- 1/2 Tbsp. Olive oil (60 calories, 0g protein, 0g carbs, 7g fat)

- Juice of 1/2 lemon (2 calories, 0g protein, 1g carb, 0g fat)

- 1/2 cup cooked quinoa (111 calories, 4g protein, 20g carbs, 2g fat)

- 10 roasted Brussels sprouts (50 calories, 3g protein, 9g carbs, 2g fat)

- Directions: Brush salmon with olive oil and bake at 400F for 10-12 minutes until cooked through. Squeeze lemon juice over top. Make quinoa according to package directions. Toss Brussels sprouts with oil, salt and pepper and roast at 425F for 15-20 minutes until browned and tender.

Day 3 Totals: Calories - 1264, Protein - 88g, Carbs - 175g, Fat - 43g

Day 4

Breakfast - Avocado Toast

- 2 slices whole wheat bread (140 calories, 8g protein, 24g carbs, 2g fat)

- 1/2 avocado, mashed (114 calories, 2g protein, 8g carbs, 10g fat)

- 1 fried egg (90 calories, 6g protein, 0g carbs, 7g fat)

- Everything but the Bagel seasoning (optional)

- Directions: Toast bread to desired crispness. Scoop out avocado flesh into bowl and mash with a fork. Spread over toast. Fry egg and top avocado toast with egg. Sprinkle with seasoning if desired.

Snack 1 - Whole Grain Crackers and Cheese

- 10 whole grain crackers (250 calories, 5g protein, 50g carbs, 1g fat per cracker)

- 1 oz cheddar cheese, cut into slices (110 calories, 7g protein, 0g carbs, 9g fat)

- Directions: Top crackers with sliced cheddar cheese.

Lunch - Grilled Chicken Caesar Salad

- 4 oz. grilled chicken breast, sliced or chopped (120 calories, 26g protein, 0g carbs, 1.5g fat)

- 2 cups chopped romaine lettuce (10 calories, 1g protein, 2g carbs, 0g fat)

- 2 Tbsp. Caesar dressing (140 calories, 0g protein, 2g carbs, 14g fat)

- 1/4 cup croutons (60 calories, 2g protein, 9g carbs, 2g fat)

- 2 Tbsp. Shredded parmesan cheese (20 calories, 2g protein, 0g carbs, 1g fat)

- Directions: Grill chicken and slice or chop. In a bowl, toss together lettuce, dressing, parmesan and croutons. Top with chicken.

Snack 2 - Trail Mix

- 1/4 cup raw almonds (200 calories, 8g protein, 6g carbs, 18g fat)

- 1/4 cup dried cranberries (140 calories, 0g protein, 32g carbs, 0g fat)

- 2 Tbsp. Pumpkin seeds (148 calories, 9g protein, 4g carbs, 12g fat)

- Directions: Combine nuts, seeds and fruit in a bowl or portable container.

Dinner - Baked Fish Tacos

- 4 oz. white fish such as cod or tilapia (120 calories, 24g protein, 0g carbs, 2g fat)

- 1 tsp chili powder (5 calories, 0g protein, 1g carb, 0g fat)

- 1 tsp cumin (8 calories, 0g protein, 0g carbs, 0g fat)

- 2 small corn tortillas (50 calories each, 1g protein, 11g carbs, 0g fat per tortilla)

- Optional toppings like salsa, cabbage slaw, avocado

- Directions: Place fish on a parchment lined baking sheet. Sprinkle with chili powder and cumin. Bake at 400F for 10-12 minutes until fish flakes easily with a fork. Serve in warmed corn tortillas with desired toppings.

Day 4 Totals: Calories - 1256, Protein - 96g, Carbs - 156g, Fat - 49g

Day 5

Breakfast - Banana Peanut Butter Protein Smoothie

- 1 medium banana (100 calories, 1g protein, 25g carbs, 0g fat)

- 1 scoop protein powder (120 calories, 25g protein, 1g carbs, 2g fat)

- 1 cup unsweetened almond milk (30 calories, 1g protein, 1g carb, 2.5g fat)

- 2 Tbsp. Natural peanut butter (190 calories, 8g protein, 6g carbs, 16g fat)

- 1 cup ice

- Directions: Add all ingredients to a high speed blender. Blend until smooth and creamy. Enjoy immediately.

Snack 1 - Greek Yogurt with Berries

- 1 cup nonfat plain Greek yogurt (100 calories, 18g protein, 9g carbs, 0g fat)

- 1/2 cup mixed berries (strawberries, blueberries, raspberries) (40 calories, 1g protein, 10g carbs, 0.5g fat)

- Directions: Spoon yogurt into a bowl. Top with fresh mixed berries.

Lunch - Turkey Burger

- 4 oz. lean ground turkey patty (140 calories, 21g protein, 1g carbs, 6g fat)

- 1 whole wheat hamburger bun (110 calories, 4g protein, 23g carbs, 1g fat)

- Lettuce, tomato, onion (optional toppings)

- 1 tsp mustard or ketchup (optional condiment)

- Directions: Grill or pan cook turkey patty over medium-high heat until no longer pink inside, about 5-7 minutes per side. Toast bun if desired. Serve patty on bun with desired condiments and toppings.

Snack 2 - Hummus and Veggies

- 3-4 Tbsp. Hummus (75-100 calories, 3-4g protein, 6-8g carbs, 5-7g fat)

- Veggies for dipping like bell pepper strips, carrots, celery, etc. (25 calories, 1g protein, 5g carbs, 0g fat)

- Directions: Arrange raw veggie dippers like bell pepper strips, carrots and celery sticks. Use hummus for dipping.

Dinner - Brown Rice and Veggie Stir Fry

- 1 cup cooked brown rice (216 calories, 5g protein, 45g carbs, 2g fat)

- 1 cup mixed stir fry veggies (broccoli, carrots, onion, bell pepper) (60 calories, 4g protein, 13g carbs, 0g fat)

- 1 Tbsp. Olive oil (119 calories, 0g protein, 0g carbs, 14g fat)

- 2 Tbsp. Reduced sodium soy sauce (10 calories, 1g protein, 1g carbs, 0g fat)

- Directions: Cook brown rice according to package directions. Heat oil in a wok or skillet over high heat. When hot, add veggies and stir fry until tender crisp, about 5 minutes. Clear center and add beaten eggs, scrambling lightly. Toss veggies and eggs together. Stir in soy sauce and serve over brown rice.

Day 5 Totals: Calories - 1260, Protein - 99g, Carbs - 165g, Fat - 49g

Day 6

Breakfast - Overnight Oats

- 1/2 cup rolled oats (150 calories, 5g protein, 27g carbs, 3g fat)

- 1/2 cup unsweetened almond milk (15 calories, 1g protein, 1g carb, 2.5g fat)

- 2 Tbsp. Chia seeds (140 calories, 5g protein, 12g carbs, 9g fat)

- 1/2 cup mixed berries like strawberries, blueberries, raspberries (40 calories, 1g protein, 10g carbs, 0.5g fat)

- 1 Tbsp. Natural peanut butter (95 calories, 4g protein, 3g carbs, 8g fat)

- Directions: In a jar or container, combine oats, chia seeds, milk and peanut butter. Stir well, cover and refrigerate overnight (or up to 2 days). Add berries before eating.

Snack 1 - Apple with Almond Butter

- 1 small apple, sliced (80 calories, 0g protein, 21g carbs, 0g fat)

- 2 Tbsp. Almond butter (180 calories, 8g protein, 6g carbs, 16g fat)

- Directions: Spread almond butter over apple slices.

Lunch - Spinach Salad with Egg and Feta

- 4 cups baby spinach (30 calories, 2g protein, 2g carbs, 0g fat)

- 1 hardboiled egg, sliced (80 calories, 6g protein, 0g carbs, 6g fat)

- 1/4 cup crumbled feta cheese (110 calories, 6g protein, 2g carbs, 9g fat)

- 2 Tbsp. balsamic vinaigrette dressing (60 calories, 0g protein, 2g carbs, 6g fat)

- Directions: In a bowl, toss together spinach, egg slices and feta cheese. Drizzle with balsamic vinaigrette right before serving.

Snack 2 - Roasted Chickpeas

- 1 15-oz can chickpeas, drained and rinsed (270 calories, 15g protein, 45g carbs, 4g fat)

- 1 Tbsp. Olive oil (119 calories, 0g protein, 0g carbs, 14g fat)

- 1/2 tsp salt

- 1/2 tsp pepper

- 1/2 tsp garlic powder

- Directions: Preheat oven to 400°F. In a bowl, toss chickpeas with oil and spices. Arrange in a single layer on a baking sheet. Roast for 20 minutes, shaking pan halfway, until browned and crispy.

Dinner - Beef and Veggie Kabobs

- 4 oz. lean beef, cubed (160 calories, 16g protein, 0g carbs, 9g fat)

- Veggies like mushrooms, onion, bell pepper, cherry tomatoes (25 calories, 2g protein, 5g carbs, 0g fat per cup veggies)

- 8 wooden or metal skewers, soaked in water for 30 minutes (0 calories)

- Marinade: 2 Tbsp. Reduced sodium soy sauce (10 calories, 1g protein, 1g carbs, 0g fat) and 1 Tbsp. Olive oil (119 calories, 0g protein, 0g carbs, 14g fat)

- Directions: In a bowl or ziploc bag, toss beef with marinade to coat. Thread beef and veggies onto skewers, alternating each. Grill over high heat, turning occasionally until beef reaches desired doneness, about 8-10 minutes for medium rare.

Day 6 Totals: Calories - 1256, Protein - 99g, Carbs - 163g, Fat - 47g

Day 7

Breakfast - Whole Grain Waffles with Peanut Butter and Banana

- 2 frozen whole grain waffles (200 calories, 5g protein, 36g carbs, 3g fat)

- 2 Tbsp. Natural peanut butter (190 calories, 8g protein, 6g carbs, 16g fat)

- 1 sliced banana (100 calories, 1g protein, 25g carbs, 0g fat)

- Directions: Toast waffles until heated through. Top with peanut butter and sliced banana.

Snack 1 - Mixed Nuts

- 14 almonds (100 calories, 4g protein, 3g carbs, 9g fat)

- 12 cashews (90 calories, 4g protein, 9g carbs, 7g fat)

- 8 walnut halves (85 calories, 4g protein, 2g carbs, 8g fat)

- Directions: Combine nuts in a bowl or take portions in a small ziploc bag for an on-the-go snack.

Lunch - Veggie Sandwich with Hummus

- 2 slices whole wheat bread (140 calories, 8g protein, 24g carbs, 2g fat)

- 3-4 Tbsp. Hummus (75-100 calories, 3-4g protein, 6-8g carbs, 5-7g fat)

- Veggie toppings like tomato slices, cucumber, lettuce, bell pepper, etc. (25 calories, 1g protein, 5g carbs, 0g fat per cup chopped veggies)

- Directions: Spread hummus evenly on bread slices. Top with desired sliced or chopped vegetables.

Snack 2 - Protein Shake

- 1 scoop protein powder, chocolate or vanilla (120 calories, 25g protein, 1g carb, 2g fat)

- 1 cup unsweetened almond milk (30 calories, 1g protein, 1g carb, 2.5g fat)

- 1 medium banana (100 calories, 1g protein, 25g carbs, 0g fat)

- Directions: Combine ingredients in blender. Blend until smooth. Add ice as desired.

Dinner - Chicken Noodle Soup

- 4 cups low sodium chicken broth (20 calories, 2g protein, 2g carbs, 0g fat per cup)

- 3 oz. cooked shredded chicken breast (140 calories, 27g protein, 0g carbs, 3g fat)

- 1 cup mixed veggies like carrots, celery, onion, etc. (30 calories, 2g protein, 7g carbs, 0g fat)

- 1 cup whole wheat noodles, dry (200 calories, 8g protein, 44g carbs, 1g fat)

- Salt, pepper and other seasonings to taste

- Directions: In a pot, bring broth to a boil. Add chicken, vegetables, noodles and seasonings. Reduce heat and simmer until noodles are tender, about 8-10 minutes.

Day 7 Totals: Calories - 1270, Protein - 102g, Carbs - 192g, Fat - 51g

Day 8

Breakfast - Breakfast Tacos

- 3 small corn tortillas (150 calories, 3g protein, 33g carbs, 1.5g fat total)

- 2 eggs scrambled (140 calories, 12g protein, 0g carbs, 10g fat)

- 1/4 cup black beans, warmed (60 calories, 3g protein, 10g carbs, 0g fat)

- 2 Tbsp. salsa (10 calories, 0g protein, 2g carbs, 0g fat)

- Hot sauce like Cholula or Tapatio (optional)

- Directions: Warm tortillas in microwave or skillet. Scramble eggs and season with a pinch of salt and pepper. Warm beans on stove or microwave. Assemble tacos by placing beans, eggs and salsa in tortillas. Add hot sauce if desired.

Snack 1 - Cottage Cheese with Pineapple

- 1/2 cup low fat cottage cheese (80 calories, 14g protein, 3g carbs, 1g fat)

- 1/2 cup fresh pineapple chunks (50 calories, 0g protein, 13g carbs, 0g fat)

- Directions: Spoon cottage cheese into a bowl or container. Top with pineapple chunks.

Lunch - Quinoa Tabbouleh Salad

- 1/2 cup uncooked quinoa (170 calories, 6g protein, 30g carbs, 3g fat)

- 1 cup chopped fresh parsley (10 calories, 1g protein, 2g carbs, 0g

- 1 cup diced tomato (30 calories, 1g protein, 7g carbs, 0g fat)

- 1/2 cup diced cucumber (10 calories, 0g protein, 2g carbs, 0g fat)

- 2 Tbsp. Olive oil (238 calories, 0g protein, 0g carbs, 27g fat)

- 2 Tbsp. Lemon juice (8 calories, 0g protein, 2g carbs, 0g fat)

- Salt and pepper to taste

- Directions: Cook quinoa according to package directions. Let cool slightly. In a bowl, combine quinoa, parsley, tomatoes, cucumber. Add oil, lemon juice and season with salt and pepper. Mix well.

Snack 2 - Celery with Nut Butter

- 4 celery sticks (5 calories, 0g protein, 1g carb, 0g fat)

- 1 Tbsp. Natural peanut or almond butter (95 calories, 4g protein, 3g carbs, 8g fat)

- Directions: Spread nut butter in the celery stalks. Enjoy as a crunchy, nutritious snack.

Dinner - Coconut Curry Shrimp

- 10 medium shrimp, peeled and deveined (100 calories, 20g protein, 1g carbs, 1g fat)

- 1/2 cup light coconut milk (80 calories, 1g protein, 5g carbs, 5g fat)

- 1 Tbsp. red curry paste (30 calories, 0g protein, 3g carbs, 1g fat)

- 1 cup mixed veggies like bell pepper, snap peas, onion (30 calories, 2g protein, 7g carbs, 0g fat)

- 1 cup "riced" cauliflower (25 calories, 2g protein, 5g carbs, 0g fat)

- 1 tsp olive oil (40 calories, 0g protein, 0g carbs, 4g fat)

- Directions: Heat oil in skillet over medium high heat. Add shrimp and veggies and cook for 2-3 minutes until shrimp start to turn pink. Add coconut milk and curry paste, bring to a simmer. Cook 2-3 more minutes until shrimp are cooked through. Serve over "riced" cauliflower.

Day 8 Totals: Calories - 1272, Protein - 96g, Carbs - 161g, Fat - 51g

Day 9

Breakfast - Peanut Butter Banana Smoothie

- 1 medium banana (100 calories, 1g protein, 25g carbs, 0g fat)

- 2 Tbsp. Natural peanut butter (190 calories, 8g protein, 6g carbs, 16g fat)

- 1 cup unsweetened almond milk (30 calories, 1g protein, 1g carb, 2.5g fat)

- Directions: In a blender, combine all ingredients with a handful of ice. Blend until smooth.

Snack 1 - Whole Grain Crackers and Cheese

- 10 whole grain crackers (250 calories, 5g protein, 50g carbs, 1g fat per cracker)

- 1 oz cheddar cheese, sliced (110 calories, 7g protein, 0g carbs, 9g fat)

- Directions: Top crackers with sliced cheddar cheese.

Lunch - Grilled Veggie and Cheese Sandwich

- 2 slices whole grain bread (140 calories, 8g protein, 24g carbs, 2g fat per slice)

- 2 slices cheddar cheese (110 calories, 7g protein, 0g carbs, 9g fat per slice)

- 1/4 cup grilled veggies like zucchini, eggplant, bell peppers, etc. (12 calories, 1g protein, 2g carbs, 0g fat)

- 1 tsp olive oil or melted butter (optional) (40 calories, 0g protein, 0g carbs, 4g fat per tsp)

- Directions: Spread one side of each bread slice with oil or butter (optional). Assemble sandwich with cheese slices and grilled veggies. Grill in panini press or skillet until golden brown and cheese is melted.

Snack 2 - Apple with Sunflower Seed Butter

- 1 small apple, sliced (80 calories, 0g protein, 21g carbs, 0g fat)

- 2 Tbsp. Sunflower seed butter (190 calories, 6g protein, 6g carbs, 16g fat)

- Directions: Spread sunflower seed butter over apple slices. Enjoy as crunchy snack.

Dinner - Roasted Pork Tenderloin

- 4 oz. pork tenderloin, trimmed (120 calories, 25g protein, 0g carbs, 2.5g fat)

- 1 tsp olive oil (40 calories, 0g protein, 0g carbs, 4g fat)

- 1/4 tsp each: garlic powder, paprika, salt

- 1 cup roasted sweet potato chunks (180 calories, 4g protein, 41g carbs, 0g fat)

- 1 cup roasted green beans (40 calories, 2g protein, 8g carbs, 0g fat)

- Directions: Rub pork tenderloin with oil and seasonings. Roast at 425F for 15-20 minutes until thermometer reads 145F. Roast sweet potato tossed in oil at same time. Roast green beans with salt and pepper. Slice pork and serve with sides.

Day 9 Totals: Calories - 1261, Protein - 69g, Carbs - 184g, Fat - 51g

Day 10

Breakfast - Yogurt Parfait with Granola and Berries

- 1 cup nonfat Greek yogurt (100 calories, 18g protein, 9g carbs, 0g fat)

- 1/2 cup mixed berries (40 calories, 1g protein, 10g carbs, 0.5g fat)

- 2 Tbsp. granola (60 calories, 1g protein, 11g carbs, 1g fat)

- Directions: In a bowl or jar, layer yogurt, berries and granola. Enjoy immediately or refrigerate overnight.

Snack 1 - Trail Mix

- 10 almonds (80 calories, 3g protein, 2g carbs, 7g fat)

- 10 cashews (75 calories, 3g protein, 7g carbs, 6g fat)

- 2 Tbsp. raisins (60 calories, 0g protein, 15g carbs, 0g fat)

- Directions: Combine nut and fruit ingredients in a bowl or portable container for easy snacking.

Lunch - Chicken Caesar Wrap

- 1 whole wheat tortilla (100 calories, 4g protein, 18g carbs, 1g fat)

- 3 oz. grilled chicken breast, sliced or chopped (105 calories, 22g protein, 0g carbs, 2g fat)

- 2 Tbsp. light Caesar dressing (80 calories, 0g protein, 1g carbs, 8g fat)

- 1/4 cup chopped romaine lettuce (2 calories, 0g protein, 0g carbs, 0g fat)

- 2 Tbsp. grated parmesan cheese (20 calories, 2g protein, 0g carbs, 1g fat)

- Directions: Place chicken, lettuce, dressing and cheese into tortilla. Roll up burrito-style to enclose fillings.

Dinner - Chili over Baked Potatoes

- 1 small baked russet potato (160 calories, 4g protein, 36g carbs, 0g fat)

- 1/2 cup chili with meat and beans (130 calories, 10g protein, 9g carbs, 7g fat)

- 2 Tbsp. shredded cheddar cheese (60 calories, 4g protein, 0g carbs, 5g fat)

- 2 Tbsp. light sour cream (30 calories, 0g protein, 2g carbs, 3g fat)

- Directions: Bake potato until tender, about 45 minutes at 425F. Split open and top with chili, cheese and sour cream.

Snack 2 - Roasted Chickpeas

- 1 15-oz can chickpeas, drained and rinsed (270 calories, 15g protein, 45g carbs, 4g fat)

- 1 Tbsp. olive oil (119 calories, 0g protein, 0g carbs, 14g fat)

- 1/2 tsp garlic powder

- 1/2 tsp smoked paprika

- 1/2 tsp sea salt

- Directions: Toss chickpeas with oil and seasonings. Roast on a baking sheet at 400F for 20 minutes, shaking halfway, until crispy.

Day 10 Totals: Calories - 1257, Protein - 85g, Carbs - 169g, Fat - 51g

Day 11

Breakfast - Veggie Omelet with Toast

- 2 eggs (140 calories, 12g protein, 0g carbs, 10g fat)

- 1/4 cup diced onion and bell pepper (15 calories, 1g protein, 3g carbs, 0g fat)

- 2 Tbsp. shredded cheddar cheese (50 calories, 4g protein, 0g carbs, 4g fat)

- 1 slice whole wheat toast (70 calories, 4g protein, 12g carbs, 1g fat)

- Directions: Whisk eggs in bowl. Heat nonstick skillet over medium heat, spray with cooking spray. Add onion and pepper, cook until softened. Pour in eggs. When eggs start to set, top with cheese. Fold omelet over and continue cooking until set. Serve with whole wheat toast.

Snack 1 - Hard Boiled Egg

- 1 large egg (80 calories, 6g protein, 0g carbs, 6g fat)

- Directions: Place egg in small pot with water to cover. Bring to a boil then reduce to simmer for 12 minutes. Cool under running water and peel.

Lunch - Tuna Salad

- 3 oz. canned tuna in water (90 calories, 21g protein, 0g carbs, 1g fat)

- 2 Tbsp. plain Greek yogurt (17 calories, 2g protein, 0g carbs, 0g fat)

- 1 Tbsp. lemon juice (4 calories, 0g protein, 1g carbs, 0g fat)

- 1/4 cup diced celery (5 calories, 0g protein, 1g carb, 0g fat)

- 2 cups mixed greens (10 calories, 1g protein, 2g carbs, 0g fat)

- Directions: In a bowl, mix together tuna, yogurt, lemon juice and celery. Serve tuna salad over mixed greens.

Snack 2 - Banana with Almond Butter

- 1 medium banana, sliced (100 calories, 1g protein, 25g carbs, 0g fat)

- 1 Tbsp. almond butter (95 calories, 4g protein, 3g carbs, 8g fat)

- Directions: Spread almond butter over the banana slices. Enjoy this potassium-rich snack!

Dinner - Turkey Meatballs

- 12 frozen or homemade turkey meatballs (240 calories, 28g protein, 12g carbs, 12g fat)

- 1/2 cup whole wheat pasta, cooked (110 calories, 4g protein, 22g carbs, 1g fat)

- 1 cup steamed broccoli florets (30 calories, 2g protein, 6g carbs, 0g fat)

- 2 Tbsp. marinara sauce (20 calories, 0g protein, 4g carbs, 0g fat)

- Directions: Bake turkey meatballs according to package directions. Cook whole wheat pasta until al dente. Steam broccoli until tender. Toss everything together with marinara sauce to coat.

Day 11 Totals: Calories - 1262, Protein - 101g, Carbs - 162g, Fat - 47g

Day 12

Breakfast - Peanut Butter Overnight Oats

- 1/2 cup rolled oats (150 calories, 5g protein, 27g carbs, 3g fat)

- 1/2 cup unsweetened almond milk (15 calories, 1g protein, 1g carb, 2.5g fat)

- 1 Tbsp. chia seeds (70 calories, 2g protein, 6g carbs, 5g fat)

- 1 Tbsp. peanut butter (95 calories, 4g protein, 3g carbs, 8g fat)

- 1/2 cup mixed berries like raspberries, blueberries, strawberries (40 calories, 1g protein, 10g carbs, 0.5g fat)

- Directions: Combine oats, chia seeds, milk and peanut butter in a jar or container. Refrigerate for at least 2 hours, or overnight. Top with fresh berries before enjoying.

Snack 1 - Hard Boiled Egg

- 1 large egg (80 calories, 6g protein, 0g carbs, 6g fat)

- Directions: Place egg in small pot with water to cover. Bring to a boil, reduce to simmer 12 minutes. Cool under running water and peel.

Lunch - Beef and Veggie Kabobs with Hummus

- 4 oz. lean beef, cubed (160 calories, 16g protein, 0g carbs, 9g fat)

- Veggies like mushrooms, peppers, onion, cherry tomatoes (25 calories, 2g protein, 5g carbs, 0g fat per cup)

- 8 wooden or metal skewers (0 calories)

- 3 Tbsp. hummus (75 calories, 3g protein, 6g carbs, 5g fat)

- Directions: Soak skewers in water for 30 minutes. Thread beef and veggies onto skewers, alternating each. Grill over medium-high heat until beef is cooked to desired doneness, about 8-10 minutes for medium. Serve kabobs with hummus for dipping.

Snack 2 - Apple with Almond Butter

- 1 small apple, sliced (80 calories, 0g protein, 21g carbs, 0g fat)

- 1 Tbsp. almond butter (95 calories, 4g protein, 3g carbs, 8g fat)

- Directions: Spread almond butter over apple slices. Enjoy this nutritious snack!

Dinner - Sheet Pan Fajitas with Shrimp

- 6 medium shrimp, peeled and deveined (60 calories, 12g protein, 0g carbs, 0g fat)

- 1 bell pepper, sliced (20 calories, 1g protein, 5g carbs, 0g fat)

- 1/2 onion, sliced (15 calories, 0g protein, 4g carbs, 0g fat)

- 2 Tbsp. fajita seasoning (20 calories, 0g protein, 2g carbs, 1g fat)

- 1 15-oz can black beans, drained and rinsed (240 calories, 15g protein, 41g carbs, 1g fat)

- 1 cup brown rice, cooked (216 calories, 5g protein, 45g carbs, 2g fat)

- Optional toppings like salsa, guacamole, cheese, lettuce, etc.

- Directions: Toss shrimp, peppers and onion with fajita seasoning. Roast at 425F for 10-12 minutes until cooked through. Serve over rice and beans with desired toppings.

Day 12 Totals: Calories - 1261, Protein - 74g, Carbs - 175g, Fat - 44g

Day 13

Breakfast - Spinach and Mushroom Omelet

- 2 eggs (140 calories, 12g protein, 0g carbs, 10g fat)

- 1/4 cup sliced mushrooms (5 calories, 1g protein, 1g carbs, 0g fat)

- 1/4 cup fresh spinach, chopped (5 calories, 1g protein, 1g carb, 0g fat)

- 1 Tbsp. feta cheese, crumbled (35 calories, 2g protein, 0g carbs, 3g fat)

- Directions: Whisk eggs in a small bowl. Heat nonstick skillet over medium heat and coat with cooking spray. Add mushrooms and spinach; sauté 1-2 minutes until softened. Pour in eggs. Cook, stirring occasionally, until set. Top with feta.

Snack 1 - Edamame

- 1/2 cup shelled edamame (95 calories, 8g protein, 8g carbs, 4g fat)

- Directions: Boil or steam edamame pods for 3-5 minutes until heated through. Sprinkle with salt if desired.

Lunch - Quinoa Chickpea Salad

- 1/2 cup cooked quinoa (111 calories, 4g protein, 20g carbs, 2g fat)

- 1/2 cup chickpeas, rinsed and drained (110 calories, 7g protein, 20g carbs, 2g fat)

- 1/4 cup chopped cucumber (5 calories, 0g protein, 1g carb, 0g fat)

- 1/4 cup halved grape tomatoes (10 calories, 0g protein, 2g carbs, 0g fat)

- 1 Tbsp. olive oil (119 calories, 0g protein, 0g carbs, 14g fat)

- 1 Tbsp. red wine vinegar (5 calories, 0g protein, 1g carb, 0g fat)

- Salt and pepper to taste

- Directions: In a bowl, combine quinoa, chickpeas, cucumber and tomatoes. Add oil and vinegar, season with salt and pepper. Stir well to coat evenly.

Snack 2 - Kale Chips

- 4 cups torn kale leaves (40 calories, 4g protein, 8g carbs, 0g fat)

- 1 Tbsp. olive oil (119 calories, 0g protein, 0g carbs, 14g fat)

- Sea salt to taste

- Directions: Tear kale into bite sized pieces, discarding thick stems. Toss with oil and salt. Bake at 375F for 5 minutes until crisp.

Dinner - Veggie Chili over Baked Potato

- 1 medium baked potato (160 calories, 4g protein, 36g carbs, 0g fat)

- 1 cup veggie chili (130 calories, 5g protein, 15g carbs, 4g fat)

- 2 Tbsp. shredded cheddar cheese (60 calories, 4g protein, 0g carbs, 5g fat)

- 2 Tbsp. Greek yogurt (13 calories, 2g protein, 0g carbs, 0g fat)

- Directions: Bake potato at 425F for 45-60 minutes until tender. Slice open and top with chili, cheese and yogurt.

Day 13 Totals: Calories - 1266, Protein - 64g, Carbs - 172g, Fat - 52g

Day 14

Breakfast - Blueberry Protein Smoothie

- 1 cup unsweetened almond milk (30 calories, 1g protein, 1g carb, 2.5g fat)

- 1/2 cup frozen blueberries (40 calories, 1g protein, 10g carbs, 0.5g fat)

- 1 scoop protein powder (120 calories, 25g protein, 1g carb, 2g fat)

- 1 Tbsp. ground flaxseed (25 calories, 1g protein, 2g carbs, 2g fat)

- Directions: Blend all ingredients together until smooth.

Snack 1 - Carrots and Hummus

- About 6 medium carrot sticks (35 calories, 1g protein, 8g carbs, 0g fat)

- 2 Tbsp. hummus (50 calories, 2g protein, 4g carbs, 3g fat)

Lunch - Mediterranean Tuna Salad

- 1 can tuna packed in water (90 calories, 20g protein, 0g carbs, 1g fat)

- 1/4 cup diced cucumber (5 calories, 0g protein, 1g carbs, 0g fat)

- 10 halved cherry tomatoes (20 calories, 1g protein, 5g carbs, 0g fat)

- 1/4 cup diced red onion (15 calories, 0g protein, 4g carbs, 0g fat)

- 1 Tbsp. olive oil (119 calories, 0g protein, 0g carbs, 14g fat)

- 1 Tbsp. red wine vinegar (2 calories, 0g protein, 0g carbs, 0g fat)

- 2 cups mixed greens (10 calories, 1g protein, 2g carbs, 0g fat)

- Directions: In a bowl, mix tuna, veggies, olive oil and vinegar. Serve over mixed greens.

Snack 2 - Cucumber Slices with Ranch

- 1/2 large cucumber, sliced (20 calories, 1g protein, 4g carbs, 0g fat)

- 2 Tbsp. ranch dressing (140 calories, 0g protein, 1g carbs, 14g fat)

Dinner - Turkey Meatloaf with Roasted Veggies

- 4 oz lean ground turkey (120 calories, 22g protein, 0g carbs, 4g fat)

- 1/4 cup whole wheat bread crumbs (30 calories, 2g protein, 6g carbs, 0g fat)

- 1 egg white (17 calories, 3g protein, 0g carbs, 0g fat)

- 1/2 cup diced carrots, roasted (30 calories, 1g protein, 7g carbs, 0g fat)

- 1/2 cup green beans, roasted (20 calories, 2g protein, 4g carbs, 0g fat)

- Directions: Mix turkey, breadcrumbs and egg. Form into a loaf and bake at 375F for 30 minutes. Toss carrots and green beans in 1 tsp oil each. Roast at 425F for 20 minutes.

Day 14 Totals: Calories - 1253, Protein - 96g, Carbs - 153g, Fat - 51g

Day 15

Breakfast - Avocado Toast with Fried Egg

- 2 slices whole wheat toast (140 calories, 8g protein, 24g carbs, 2g fat)

- 1/2 avocado, mashed (114 calories, 2g protein, 8g carbs, 10g fat)

- 1 fried egg (90 calories, 6g protein, 0g carbs, 7g fat)

- Everything bagel seasoning (optional)

- Directions: Toast bread. Mash avocado on top and add fried egg. Sprinkle with seasoning if desired.

Snack 1 - Greek Yogurt with Granola

- 1 cup nonfat Greek yogurt (100 calories, 18g protein, 9g carbs, 0g fat)

- 2 Tbsp. granola (60 calories, 1g protein, 9g carbs, 1g fat)

Lunch - Grilled Chicken Pita

- 1 whole wheat pita (100 calories, 4g protein, 18g carbs, 1g fat)

- 3 oz. grilled chicken breast, diced (105 calories, 22g protein, 0g carbs, 2g fat)

- 1/4 cup chopped cucumber (5 calories, 0g protein, 1g carbs, 0g fat)

- 1/4 cup halved cherry tomatoes (10 calories, 0g protein, 2g carbs, 0g fat)

- 2 Tbsp. hummus (50 calories, 2g protein, 4g carbs, 3g fat)

- Directions: Stuff pita with chicken, veggies and hummus.

Snack 2 - Fresh Berries

- 1 cup mixed berries like strawberries, blueberries, raspberries (80 calories, 1g protein, 19g carbs, 0.5g fat)

Dinner - Baked Tilapia with Brown Rice and Broccoli

- 4 oz. tilapia fillet (100 calories, 22g protein, 0g carbs, 2g fat)

- 1/2 cup brown rice (108 calories, 2g protein, 23g carbs, 1g fat)

- 1 cup broccoli florets, steamed (30 calories, 2g protein, 6g carbs, 0g fat)

- Lemon wedges

- Directions: Bake tilapia at 400F for 10-12 minutes until flaky. Make rice according to package directions. Steam broccoli until tender. Squeeze lemon juice over fish before serving.

Day 15 Totals: Calories - 1249, Protein - 105g, Carbs - 155g, Fat - 44g

Day 16

Breakfast - Overnight Oats with Chia Seeds

- 1/2 cup rolled oats (150 calories, 5g protein, 27g carbs, 3g fat)

- 1/2 cup unsweetened almond milk (15 calories, 1g protein, 1g carb, 2.5g fat)

- 1 Tbsp. chia seeds (70 calories, 2g protein, 6g carbs, 5g fat)

- 1/2 cup mixed berries (40 calories, 1g protein, 10g carbs, 0.5g fat)

- Directions: Stir together oats, chia seeds and milk in a jar or container. Refrigerate overnight. Top with berries before eating.

Snack 1 - Cottage Cheese with Pineapple

- 1/2 cup low fat cottage cheese (80 calories, 14g protein, 3g carbs, 1g fat)

- 1/2 cup pineapple chunks (50 calories, 0g protein, 13g carbs, 0g fat)

Lunch - Lentil and Quinoa Bowl

- 1/2 cup cooked quinoa (111 calories, 4g protein, 20g carbs, 2g fat)

- 1/2 cup cooked lentils (115 calories, 9g protein, 20g carbs, 0g fat)

- 1 cup spinach (10 calories, 1g protein, 1g carbs, 0g fat)

- 1/4 avocado, sliced (60 calories, 1g protein, 3g carbs, 6g fat)

- Lemon juice (optional)

- Directions: Combine quinoa, lentils and spinach. Top with avocado and lemon juice if desired.

Snack 2 - Apple with Sunflower Seed Butter

- 1 small apple, sliced (80 calories, 0g protein, 21g carbs, 0g fat)

- 1 Tbsp. sunflower seed butter (95 calories, 4g protein, 4g carbs, 8g fat)

Dinner - Chicken Parmesan

- 4 oz. chicken breast (120 calories, 26g protein, 0g carbs, 1.5g fat)

- 2 Tbsp. marinara sauce (30 calories, 1g protein, 5g carbs, 0g fat)

- 2 Tbsp. shredded mozzarella (50 calories, 4g protein, 1g carbs, 4g fat)

- 1/2 cup whole wheat pasta (110 calories, 4g protein, 22g carbs, 1g fat)

- 1 cup steamed broccoli (30 calories, 2g protein, 6g carbs, 0g fat)

- Directions: Bread chicken breast with seasoning, bake at 400F until cooked through. Top with sauce and cheese. Serve over pasta and broccoli.

Day 16 Totals: Calories - 1256, Protein - 103g, Carbs - 166g, Fat - 42g

Day 17

Breakfast - Spinach and Goat Cheese Egg Bake

- 2 eggs (140 calories, 12g protein, 0g carbs, 10g fat)

- 1/4 cup egg whites (30 calories, 6g protein, 0g carbs, 0g fat)

- 1/4 cup spinach, chopped small (2 calories, 0g protein, 0g carbs, 0g fat)

- 1 oz. goat cheese, crumbled (75 calories, 5g protein, 0g carbs, 6g fat)

- Directions: Whisk eggs and egg whites together. Stir in spinach and goat cheese. Pour into greased ramekin dishes and bake at 350F for 20-25 minutes until set.

Snack 1 - Mixed Nuts

- 10 almonds (70 calories, 3g protein, 2g carbs, 7g fat)

- 8 cashews (60 calories, 3g protein, 5g carbs, 5g fat)

- 2 Brazil nuts (45 calories, 1g protein, 1g carbs, 4g fat)

Lunch - Salmon Burger with Sweet Potato Fries

- 1 salmon burger patty (130 calories, 15g protein, 4g carbs, 6g fat)

- 10 oven baked sweet potato fries (120 calories, 2g protein, 20g carbs, 4g fat)

- Directions: Bake salmon patty and sweet potato fries at 425F for 15-20 minutes, flipping halfway.

Snack 2 - Carrots and Hummus

- About 5 medium carrot sticks (25 calories, 1g protein, 6g carbs, 0g fat)

- 2 Tbsp. hummus (50 calories, 2g protein, 4g carbs, 3g fat)

Dinner - Veggie Fried Rice

- 1 cup "riced" cauliflower (25 calories, 2g protein, 5g carbs, 0g fat)

- 1/2 cup peas and carrots blend (60 calories, 3g protein, 11g carbs, 0g fat)

- 1 Tbsp. olive oil (119 calories, 0g protein, 0g carbs, 14g fat)

- 1 egg, scrambled (70 calories, 6g protein, 0g carbs, 5g fat)

- 1 Tbsp. reduced sodium soy sauce (5 calories, 1g protein, 1g carb, 0g fat)

- Directions: Prepare riced cauliflower. Heat oil in pan. Add veggies and stir fry until tender. Push veggies to side, pour beaten egg into pan and scramble. Toss everything together and stir in soy sauce.

Day 17 Totals: Calories - 1256, Protein - 89g, Carbs - 140g, Fat - 51g

Day 18

Breakfast - Berry Smoothie Bowl

- 1 cup frozen mixed berries (blueberries, strawberries, raspberries) (80 calories, 1g protein, 19g carbs, 0.5g fat)

- 1 banana (100 calories, 1g protein, 25g carbs, 0g fat)

- 1/2 cup nonfat Greek yogurt (50 calories, 9g protein, 5g carbs, 0g fat)

- 1 Tbsp. chopped walnuts (50 calories, 2g protein, 2g carbs, 5g fat)

- Directions: Blend berries, banana and yogurt. Top with nuts.

Snack 1 - Hard Boiled Egg

- 1 large egg (80 calories, 6g protein, 0g carbs, 6g fat)

Lunch - Chicken Caesar Salad Wrap

- 1 whole wheat tortilla (100 calories, 4g protein, 18g carbs, 1g fat)

- 3 oz. grilled chicken, chopped (105 calories, 22g protein, 0g carbs, 2g fat)

- 2 cups chopped romaine (10 calories, 1g protein, 2g carbs, 0g fat)

- 2 Tbsp. light Caesar dressing (70 calories, 0g protein, 1g carbs, 7g fat)

- Directions: Spread dressing on tortilla, top with chicken and lettuce. Roll up to make a wrap.

Snack 2 - Greek Yogurt with Granola

- 1 cup nonfat Greek yogurt (100 calories, 18g protein, 9g carbs, 0g fat)

- 2 Tbsp. granola (60 calories, 1g protein, 9g carbs, 1g fat)

Dinner - Beef and Broccoli Stir Fry

- 4 oz. flank steak, sliced thin (240 calories, 24g protein, 0g carbs, 12g fat)

- 1 cup broccoli florets (30 calories, 2g protein, 6g carbs, 0g fat)

- 1 Tbsp. reduced sodium soy sauce (5 calories, 1g protein, 1g carb, 0g fat)

- 1 tsp sesame oil (40 calories, 0g protein, 0g carbs, 4g fat)

- 1 cup brown rice (216 calories, 5g protein, 45g carbs, 2g fat)

- Directions: Stir fry beef and broccoli in small amounts of water until beef is cooked and broccoli is tender. Toss with soy sauce and sesame oil. Serve over brown rice.

Day 18 Totals: Calories - 1256, Protein - 106g, Carbs - 160g, Fat - 43g

Day 19

Breakfast - Tofu Veggie Scramble

- 1/2 block firm tofu, drained and crumbled (150 calories, 16g protein, 4g carbs, 8g fat)

- 1/4 cup diced onion (15 calories, 0g protein, 4g carbs, 0g fat)

- 1/4 cup diced bell pepper (10 calories, 0g protein, 2g carbs, 0g fat)

- 1/2 tsp turmeric

- 1/4 tsp garlic powder

- Salt and pepper to taste

- Directions: Sauté tofu and veggies until softened. Season with spices.

Snack 1 - Roasted Chickpeas

- 1 15-oz can chickpeas, drained and rinsed (270 calories, 15g protein, 45g carbs, 4g fat)

- 1 Tbsp. olive oil (119 calories, 0g protein, 0g carbs, 14g fat)

- 1/2 tsp smoked paprika

- 1/4 tsp garlic powder

- Directions: Toss chickpeas with oil and spices. Roast at 400F for 20 minutes, shaking pan halfway.

Lunch - Falafel Pita

- 4-5 baked or fried falafel patties (240 calories, 12g protein, 33g carbs, 7g fat)

- 1 whole wheat pita (100 calories, 4g protein, 18g carbs, 1g fat)

- 1/4 cup chopped tomatoes (5 calories, 0g protein, 1g carbs, 0g fat)

- 1/4 cup cucumbers, sliced (5 calories, 0g protein, 1g carbs, 0g fat)

- 2-3 Tbsp. hummus (50 calories, 2g protein, 4g carbs, 3g fat)

- Directions: Stuff pita with falafel patties, tomatoes, cucumbers and hummus.

Snack 2 - Apple with Almond Butter

- 1 small apple, sliced (80 calories, 0g protein, 21g carbs, 0g fat)

- 1 Tbsp. almond butter (90 calories, 4g protein, 3g carbs, 8g fat)

Dinner - Fish Tacos with Cabbage Slaw

- 4 oz. tilapia or cod (120 calories, 24g protein, 0g carbs, 2g fat)

- 2 corn tortillas (50 calories each, 1g protein, 11g carbs, 0g fat per tortilla)

- 1/2 cup cabbage slaw (15 calories, 0g protein, 4g carbs, 0g fat)

- 1 Tbsp. salsa (5 calories, 0g protein, 1g carb, 0g fat)

- Lime wedge

- Directions: Bake fish coated in spices. Assemble tacos with cabbage slaw, salsa and lime juice.

Day 19 Totals: Calories - 1249, Protein - 102g, Carbs - 181g, Fat - 46g

Day 20

Breakfast - Overnight Oats with Peanut Butter

- 1/2 cup rolled oats (150 calories, 5g protein, 27g carbs, 3g fat)

- 1/2 cup unsweetened almond milk (15 calories, 1g protein, 1g carb, 2.5g fat)

- 1 Tbsp. peanut butter (95 calories, 4g protein, 3g carbs, 8g fat)

- 1/2 medium banana, sliced (50 calories, 1g protein, 13g carbs, 0g fat)

- Directions: Combine oats, milk and peanut butter in a jar. Refrigerate overnight. Top with banana before eating.

Snack 1 - Edamame

- 1/2 cup shelled edamame (95 calories, 8g protein, 9g carbs, 4g fat)

- Directions: Cook frozen edamame according to package instructions until heated through.

Lunch - Quinoa Tabbouleh Salad with Tuna

- 1/2 cup cooked quinoa (111 calories, 4g protein, 20g carbs, 2g fat)

- 3 oz. canned tuna (90 calories, 21g protein, 0g carbs, 1g fat)

- 1/4 cup diced tomatoes (10 calories, 0g protein, 2g carbs, 0g fat)

- 1/4 cup diced cucumber (5 calories, 0g protein, 1g carbs, 0g fat)

- 1 Tbsp. lemon juice (4 calories, 0g protein, 1g carbs, 0g fat)

- 1 Tbsp. olive oil (119 calories, 0g protein, 0g carbs, 14g fat)

- Directions: Mix quinoa, tuna, tomatoes, cucumber, lemon juice and olive oil. Chill until ready to eat.

Snack 2 - Trail Mix

- 10 almonds (70 calories, 3g protein, 2g carbs, 7g fat)

- 10 cashews (75 calories, 3g protein, 7g carbs, 6g fat)

- 1 Tbsp. raisins (30 calories, 0g protein, 8g carbs, 0g fat)

Dinner - Baked Ziti with Turkey Sausage

- 2 oz. dry whole wheat ziti, cooked (200 calories, 8g protein, 40g carbs, 1g fat)

- 3 oz. Italian turkey sausage (150 calories, 15g protein, 1g carbs, 12g fat)

- 1/2 cup marinara sauce (60 calories, 2g protein, 10g carbs, 1g fat)

- 2 Tbsp. shredded mozzarella (50 calories, 4g protein, 1g carbs, 4g fat)

- Directions: Cook ziti according to package directions. Brown sausage, then combine with pasta, sauce and cheese. Bake at 350F for 20 minutes.

Day 20 Totals: Calories - 1255, Protein - 100g, Carbs - 164g, Fat - 47g

Day 21

Breakfast - Protein Pancakes

- 1/4 cup protein powder (120 calories, 25g protein, 1g carb, 2g fat)

- 1/4 cup egg whites (60 calories, 12g protein, 0g carbs, 0g fat)

- 1/4 cup oats (75 calories, 3g protein, 13g carbs, 2g fat)

- 1 tsp baking powder

- 1/4 tsp cinnamon

- 1 tsp vanilla extract

- 1/4 cup milk of choice

- Directions: Mix all ingredients until combined. Pour batter into greased pan and cook like regular pancakes.

Snack 1 - Cottage Cheese and Berries

- 1/2 cup low fat cottage cheese (80 calories, 14g protein, 3g carbs, 1g fat)

- 1/2 cup mixed berries (40 calories, 1g protein, 10g carbs, 0.5g fat)

Lunch - Chicken Pesto Sandwich

- 2 slices whole wheat bread (140 calories, 8g protein, 24g carbs, 2g fat)

- 3 oz. cooked chicken breast, sliced (105 calories, 22g protein, 0g carbs, 2g fat)

- 2 Tbsp. pesto (80 calories, 1g protein, 2g carbs, 8g fat)

- Lettuce, tomato, onion (optional)

- Directions: Spread pesto on bread. Top with chicken and veggies.

Snack 2 - Cucumber Slices with Hummus

- 1/2 large cucumber, sliced (20 calories, 1g protein, 4g carbs, 0g fat)

- 2 Tbsp. hummus (50 calories, 2g protein, 4g carbs, 3g fat)

Dinner - Lemon Pepper Cod with Rice and Spinach

- 4 oz. cod fillet (120 calories, 24g protein, 0g carbs, 1g fat)

- 1 tsp olive oil (40 calories, 0g protein, 0g carbs, 4g fat)

- 1/2 tsp lemon pepper seasoning

- 1/2 cup brown rice (108 calories, 2g protein, 23g carbs, 1g fat)

- 1 cup steamed spinach (30 calories, 2g protein, 6g carbs, 0g fat)

- Lemon wedge

- Directions: Coat cod in oil and seasoning. Bake at 400F for 10-12 minutes until flaky. Serve over rice and spinach. Squeeze lemon over top.

Day 21 Totals: Calories - 1248, Protein - 113g, Carbs - 151g, Fat - 41g

Day 22

Breakfast - Breakfast Taco

- 1 corn tortilla (50 calories, 1g protein, 11g carbs, 0g fat)

- 1 scrambled egg (70 calories, 6g protein, 0g carbs, 5g fat)

- 1 Tbsp. shredded cheddar cheese (25 calories, 2g protein, 0g carbs, 2g fat)

- 2 Tbsp. salsa (10 calories, 0g protein, 2g carbs, 0g fat)

- Directions: Warm the tortilla. Scramble egg and top with cheese and salsa. Roll up taco style.

Snack 1 - Carrots with Ranch Dip

- 5-6 baby carrots (30 calories, 1g protein, 7g carbs, 0g fat)

- 2 Tbsp. ranch dressing (140 calories, 0g protein, 1g carbs, 14g fat)

Lunch - Chopped Chef Salad

- 2 cups chopped romaine lettuce (10 calories, 1g protein, 2g carbs, 0g fat)

- 2 oz. chopped deli turkey (60 calories, 13g protein, 1g carbs, 1g fat)

- 2 Tbsp. shredded cheddar cheese (50 calories, 4g protein, 1g carbs, 4g fat)

- 5 grape tomatoes, halved (10 calories, 0g protein, 2g carbs, 0g fat)

- 1 Tbsp. ranch dressing (70 calories, 0g protein, 1g carb, 7g fat)

- Directions: Toss together lettuce, turkey, cheese and tomatoes. Drizzle with ranch.

Snack 2 - Mixed Nuts

- 10 almonds (70 calories, 3g protein, 2g carbs, 7g fat)

- 5 cashews (40 calories, 2g protein, 3g carbs, 3g fat)

- 5 pecan halves (90 calories, 1g protein, 4g carbs, 9g fat)

Dinner - Veggie and Chickpea Curry

- 1/2 cup chickpeas (100 calories, 5g protein, 14g carbs, 0g fat)

- 1 cup cauliflower florets (30 calories, 2g protein, 5g carbs, 0g fat)

- 1/2 cup diced tomato (15 calories, 0g protein, 4g carbs, 0g fat)

- 1/2 cup peas (60 calories, 4g protein, 10g carbs, 0g fat)

- 1 Tbsp. olive oil (119 calories, 0g protein, 0g carbs, 14g fat)

- 1 Tbsp. curry powder

- 1 cup cooked brown rice (216 calories, 5g protein, 45g carbs, 2g fat)

- Directions: Sauté chickpeas, cauliflower, tomato and spices in oil. Serve curry over brown rice.

Day 22 Totals: Calories - 1246, Protein - 71g, Carbs - 177g, Fat - 45g

Day 23

Breakfast - Berry Smoothie

- 1 cup frozen mixed berries (80 calories, 1g protein, 19g carbs, 0.5g fat)

- 1 banana (100 calories, 1g protein, 25g carbs, 0g fat)

- 1 cup unsweetened almond milk (30 calories, 1g protein, 1g carb, 2.5g fat)

- 1 scoop protein powder (optional) (120 calories, 25g protein, 1g carb, 2g fat)

- Directions: Blend all ingredients until smooth and creamy.

Snack 1 - Hard Boiled Egg

- 1 large egg (80 calories, 6g protein, 0g carbs, 6g fat)

Lunch - Grilled Chicken Pita

- 1 whole wheat pita (100 calories, 4g protein, 18g carbs, 1g fat)

- 3 oz. grilled chicken breast, diced (105 calories, 22g protein, 0g carbs, 2g fat)

- Lettuce, tomato, cucumbers (optional fillings)

- 2 Tbsp. hummus (50 calories, 2g protein, 4g carbs, 3g fat)

- Directions: Stuff pita with chicken, veggies and hummus.

Snack 2 - Apple with Peanut Butter

- 1 small apple, sliced (80 calories, 0g protein, 21g carbs, 0g fat)

- 1 Tbsp. peanut butter (95 calories, 4g protein, 3g carbs, 8g fat)

Dinner - Spaghetti Squash Bolognese

- 1 cup cooked spaghetti squash (42 calories, 1g protein, 10g carbs, 0g fat)

- 1/2 cup turkey meat sauce (150 calories, 15g protein, 8g carbs, 7g fat)

- 2 Tbsp. shredded parmesan cheese (20 calories, 2g protein, 0g carbs, 1g fat)

- Directions: Make spaghetti squash noodles and turkey meat sauce. Top squash with sauce and parmesan.

Day 23 Totals: Calories - 1252, Protein - 94g, Carbs - 157g, Fat - 43g

Day 24

Breakfast - Veggie Omelet

- 2 eggs (140 calories, 12g protein, 0g carbs, 10g fat)

- 1/4 cup diced bell pepper (10 calories, 0g protein, 2g carbs, 0g fat)

- 1/4 cup diced onion (15 calories, 0g protein, 4g carbs, 0g fat)

- 2 Tbsp. shredded cheddar cheese (50 calories, 4g protein, 0g carbs, 4g fat)

- Directions: Whisk eggs, add veggies. Cook eggs until set, sprinkle cheese on top.

Snack 1 - Greek Yogurt with Granola

- 1 cup nonfat Greek yogurt (100 calories, 18g protein, 9g carbs, 0g fat)

- 2 Tbsp. granola (60 calories, 1g protein, 9g carbs, 1g fat)

Lunch - Salmon Salad

- 3 oz. canned salmon (90 calories, 19g protein, 0g carbs, 3g fat)

- 2 cups mixed greens (10 calories, 1g protein, 2g carbs, 0g fat)

- 1/4 cup cherry tomatoes (10 calories, 0g protein, 2g carbs, 0g fat)

- 1 Tbsp. balsamic vinaigrette (45 calories, 0g protein, 1g carbs, 5g fat)

- Directions: Toss greens, tomatoes and dressing. Top with salmon.

Snack 2 - Kale Chips

- 2 cups torn kale leaves (20 calories, 2g protein, 4g carbs, 0g fat)

- 1 tsp olive oil (40 calories, 0g protein, 0g carbs, 4g fat)

- Sea salt to taste

- Directions: Toss kale with oil and salt. Bake at 375F for 5 minutes until crispy.

Dinner - Pork Chops with Roasted Veggies

- 4 oz. boneless pork chop (180 calories, 26g protein, 0g carbs, 8g fat)

- 1/2 cup roasted potatoes (50 calories, 1g protein, 12g carbs, 0g fat)

- 1/2 cup roasted carrots (25 calories, 1g protein, 6g carbs, 0g fat)

- Directions: Brush pork chop with oil and seasoning of choice. Roast at 400F for 15 minutes until cooked through. Toss potatoes and carrots in oil, roast at 425F until browned and tender.

Day 24 Totals: Calories - 1245, Protein - 104g, Carbs - 132g, Fat - 47g

Day 25

Breakfast - Overnight Oats with Chia Seeds

- 1/2 cup rolled oats (150 calories, 5g protein, 27g carbs, 3g fat)

- 1/2 cup unsweetened almond milk (15 calories, 1g protein, 1g carb, 2.5g fat)

- 1 Tbsp. chia seeds (70 calories, 2g protein, 6g carbs, 5g fat)

- Directions: Stir together oats, chia seeds and milk in a jar or container. Refrigerate overnight.

Snack 1 - Hummus and Carrots

- About 5 carrot sticks (25 calories, 1g protein, 6g carbs, 0g fat)

- 2 Tbsp. hummus (50 calories, 2g protein, 4g carbs, 3g fat)

Lunch - Burrito Bowl

- 1/2 cup rice (103 calories, 2g protein, 22g carbs, 0g fat)

- 1/2 cup black beans (120 calories, 8g protein, 20g carbs, 1g fat)

- 3 oz. shredded chicken (105 calories, 22g protein, 0g carbs, 2g fat)

- 1/4 cup salsa (10 calories, 0g protein, 2g carbs, 0g fat)

- 2 Tbsp. shredded cheese (optional) (50 calories, 4g protein, 1g carb, 4g fat)

- Directions: Assemble rice, beans, chicken and desired toppings in a bowl.

Snack 2 - Fresh Berries

- 1 cup mixed berries (80 calories, 1g protein, 19g carbs, 0.5g fat)

Dinner - Pasta with Meatballs and Broccoli

- 1/2 cup whole wheat pasta (110 calories, 4g protein, 22g carbs, 1g fat)

- 4 frozen or homemade meatballs (200 calories, 12g protein, 10g carbs, 14g fat)

- 1 cup broccoli florets, steamed (30 calories, 2g protein, 6g carbs, 0g fat)

- 2 Tbsp. marinara sauce (30 calories, 1g protein, 5g carbs, 0g fat)

- Directions: Cook pasta according to package directions. Bake meatballs. Steam broccoli until tender. Toss everything with marinara sauce.

Day 25 Totals: Calories - 1249, Protein - 94g, Carbs - 166g, Fat - 43g

Day 26

Breakfast - Peanut Butter Toast with Banana

- 2 slices whole wheat bread (140 calories, 8g protein, 24g carbs, 2g fat)

- 2 Tbsp. peanut butter (190 calories, 8g protein, 6g carbs, 16g fat)

- 1 medium banana, sliced (100 calories, 1g protein, 25g carbs, 0g fat)

- Directions: Toast bread if desired. Spread peanut butter on toast and top with sliced banana.

Snack 1 - Cottage Cheese and Pineapple

- 1/2 cup low fat cottage cheese (80 calories, 14g protein, 3g carbs, 1g fat)

- 1/2 cup pineapple chunks (50 calories, 0g protein, 13g carbs, 0g fat)

Lunch - Chopped Kale Salad with Chicken

- 2 cups chopped kale (20 calories, 2g protein, 4g carbs, 0g fat)

- 3 oz. cooked chicken breast, chopped (105 calories, 22g protein, 0g carbs, 2g fat)

- 1/4 cup dried cranberries (140 calories, 0g protein, 32g carbs, 0g fat)

- 1 Tbsp. balsamic vinaigrette (45 calories, 0g protein, 1g carbs, 5g fat)

- Directions: Toss together kale, chicken, cranberries and dressing.

Snack 2 - Apple with Sunflower Seed Butter

- 1 small apple, sliced (80 calories, 0g protein, 21g carbs, 0g fat)

- 1 Tbsp. sunflower seed butter (95 calories, 4g protein, 4g carbs, 8g fat)

Dinner - Fish Tacos with Cauliflower Rice

- 4 oz. tilapia or cod (120 calories, 24g protein, 0g carbs, 2g fat)

- 1 cup "riced" cauliflower (25 calories, 2g protein, 5g carbs, 0g fat)

- 1 Tbsp. salsa (5 calories, 0g protein, 1g carb, 0g fat)

- 1 corn tortilla (50 calories, 1g protein, 11g carbs, 0g fat)

- Lime wedge

- Directions: Bake fish coated in spices. Assemble tacos with fish, cauliflower rice, salsa and lime juice.

Day 26 Totals: Calories - 1250, Protein - 101g, Carbs - 178g, Fat - 47g

Day 27

Breakfast - Spinach and Mushroom Omelet

- 2 eggs (140 calories, 12g protein, 0g carbs, 10g fat)

- 1/4 cup spinach, roughly chopped (3 calories, 0g protein, 1g carbs, 0g fat)

- 1/4 cup sliced mushrooms (5 calories, 1g protein, 1g carbs, 0g fat)

- 2 Tbsp. shredded cheddar cheese (50 calories, 4g protein, 0g carbs, 4g fat)

- Directions: Whisk eggs, add spinach and mushrooms. Cook eggs until set, sprinkle cheese on top.

Snack 1 - Roasted Chickpeas

- 1 15-oz can chickpeas, drained and rinsed (270 calories, 15g protein, 45g carbs, 4g fat)

- 1 Tbsp. olive oil (119 calories, 0g protein, 0g carbs, 14g fat)

- 1/2 tsp garlic powder

- 1/2 tsp onion powder

- Directions: Toss chickpeas in oil and spices. Roast at 400F for 20 minutes, shaking pan halfway.

Lunch - Lentil Soup

- 1/2 cup dried lentils (230 calories, 17g protein, 40g carbs, 1g fat)

- 1 small onion, diced (40 calories, 1g protein, 9g carbs, 0g fat)

- 2 carrots, diced (35 calories, 1g protein, 8g carbs, 0g fat)

- 4 cups low sodium vegetable broth (20 calories, 2g protein, 2g carbs, 0g fat per cup)

- 1 bay leaf

- Salt and pepper to taste

- Directions: Simmer lentils and vegetables in broth until soft, about 30 minutes. Season with salt and pepper.

Snack 2 - Carrots and Ranch Dip

- About 5 medium carrot sticks (25 calories, 1g protein, 6g carbs, 0g fat)

- 2 Tbsp. ranch dressing (140 calories, 0g protein, 1g carbs, 14g fat)

Dinner - Stuffed Peppers

- 1 large bell pepper (30 calories, 1g protein, 7g carbs, 0g fat)

- 4 oz. lean ground turkey (120 calories, 22g protein, 0g carbs, 4g fat)

- 1/4 cup brown rice (54 calories, 1g protein, 12g carbs, 0g fat)

- 1 Tbsp. taco seasoning

- 2 Tbsp. shredded cheddar cheese (topping) (50 calories, 4g protein, 1g carb, 4g fat)

- Directions: Brown turkey with taco seasoning. Fill pepper with turkey mixture, top with cheese. Bake at 375F for 25 minutes.

Day 27 Totals: Calories - 1249, Protein - 93g, Carbs - 179g, Fat - 45g

Day 28

Breakfast - Acai Bowl

- 1 packet frozen acai smoothie pack (100 calories, 1g protein, 21g carbs, 1g fat)

- 1/2 banana, sliced (50 calories, 1g protein, 13g carbs, 0g fat)

- 1/4 cup granola (110 calories, 3g protein, 18g carbs, 2g fat)

- Directions: Blend smoothie pack with banana. Top with granola.

Snack 1 - Hard Boiled Egg

- 1 large egg (80 calories, 6g protein, 0g carbs, 6g fat)

Day 28 Lunch - Chicken Pesto Panini

- 2 slices whole wheat bread (140 calories, 8g protein, 24g carbs, 2g fat)

- 3 oz grilled chicken breast, sliced (105 calories, 22g protein, 0g carbs, 2g fat)

- 1 Tbsp. pesto (40 calories, 0g protein, 1g carbs, 4g fat)

- 2 slices tomato (optional)

- Directions: Spread pesto on bread. Add chicken and tomato. Grill panini until bread is toasted and fillings warmed.

Snack 2 - Cucumber Slices with Hummus

- 1/2 large cucumber, sliced (20 calories, 1g protein, 4g carbs, 0g fat)

- 2 Tbsp. hummus (50 calories, 2g protein, 4g carbs, 3g fat)

Dinner - Shrimp Fried Rice

- 8-10 medium shrimp, peeled (70 calories, 15g protein, 0g carbs, 1g fat)

- 1 egg, beaten (70 calories, 6g protein, 0g carbs, 5g fat)

- 1/2 cup frozen peas and carrots (60 calories, 3g protein, 11g carbs, 0g fat)

- 1 cup cooked brown rice (216 calories, 5g protein, 45g carbs, 2g fat)

- 1 Tbsp. reduced sodium soy sauce (5 calories, 1g protein, 1g carb, 0g fat)

- 1 tsp sesame oil (40 calories, 0g protein, 0g carbs, 4g fat)

- Green onions, chopped (optional garnish)

- Directions: Stir fry shrimp, egg, peas and carrots. Toss with rice, soy sauce and sesame oil. Garnish with green onions.

Day 28 Totals: Calories - 1246, Protein - 90g, Carbs - 167g, Fat - 42g

Day 29

Breakfast - Breakfast Tacos

- 2 corn tortillas (100 calories, 2g protein, 22g carbs, 1g fat)

- 2 eggs, scrambled (140 calories, 12g protein, 0g carbs, 10g fat)

- 2 Tbsp. shredded cheddar cheese (50 calories, 4g protein, 1g carb, 4g fat)

- 1/4 cup black beans (30 calories, 2g protein, 5g carbs, 0g fat)

- Salsa or hot sauce (optional)

- Directions: Warm tortillas. Scramble eggs with beans and cheese. Fill tortillas.

Snack 1 - Mixed Nuts

- 10 almonds (70 calories, 3g protein, 2g carbs, 7g fat)

- 5 cashews (40 calories, 2g protein, 3g carbs, 3g fat)

- 2 Brazil nuts (45 calories, 1g protein, 1g carbs, 4g fat)

Lunch - Salmon Salad

- 3 oz. canned salmon (90 calories, 19g protein, 0g carbs, 3g fat)

- 2 cups mixed greens (10 calories, 1g protein, 2g carbs, 0g fat)

- 1/4 cup cherry tomatoes (10 calories, 0g protein, 2g carbs, 0g fat)

- 1 Tbsp. balsamic vinaigrette (45 calories, 0g protein, 1g carbs, 5g fat)

- Directions: Toss greens, tomatoes and dressing. Top with salmon.

Snack 2 - Greek Yogurt with Berries

- 1 cup nonfat Greek yogurt (100 calories, 18g protein, 9g carbs, 0g fat)

- 1/2 cup mixed berries (40 calories, 1g protein, 10g carbs, 0.5g fat)

Dinner - Tofu Veggie Stir Fry

- 1/2 block firm tofu, diced (150 calories, 16g protein, 4g carbs, 8g fat)

- 1 cup mixed stir fry veggies like broccoli, carrots, bell peppers (30 calories, 2g protein, 7g carbs, 0g fat)

- 1 Tbsp. reduced sodium soy sauce (5 calories, 1g protein, 1g carb, 0g fat)

- 1 tsp sesame oil (40 calories, 0g protein, 0g carbs, 4g fat)

- 1 cup brown rice (216 calories, 5g protein, 45g carbs, 2g fat)

- Directions: Stir fry tofu and vegetables until tender. Toss with soy sauce and sesame oil. Serve over brown rice.

Day 29 Totals: Calories - 1242, Protein - 99g, Carbs - 171g, Fat - 45g

Day 30

Breakfast - Avocado Toast with Egg

- 2 slices whole wheat toast (140 calories, 8g protein, 24g carbs, 2g fat)

- 1/2 avocado, mashed (114 calories, 2g protein, 8g carbs, 10g fat)

- 1 fried egg (90 calories, 6g protein, 0g carbs, 7g fat)

- Everything bagel seasoning (optional)

- Directions: Toast bread. Mash avocado on top. Add fried egg and sprinkle with seasoning.

Snack 1 - Edamame

- 1/2 cup shelled edamame (95 calories, 8g protein, 9g carbs, 4g fat)

- Directions: Prepare frozen edamame according to package - boil or microwave until heated through.

Lunch - Quinoa and Black Bean Bowl

- 1/2 cup cooked quinoa (111 calories, 4g protein, 20g carbs, 2g fat)

- 1/2 cup black beans, rinsed and drained (120 calories, 8g protein, 20g carbs, 1g fat)

- 1/4 avocado, diced (60 calories, 1g protein, 3g carbs, 6g fat)

- Salsa, hot sauce, chopped veggies etc. (optional toppings)

- Directions: Mix together quinoa, black beans and avocado. Add any other desired toppings.

Snack 2 - Apple with Almond Butter

- 1 small apple, sliced (80 calories, 0g protein, 21g carbs, 0g fat)

- 1 Tbsp. almond butter (90 calories, 4g protein, 3g carbs, 8g fat)

Dinner - Veggie Pizza

- 1/2 whole wheat pizza crust or flatbread (120 calories, 5g protein, 22g carbs, 1g fat)

- 1/4 cup pizza sauce (30 calories, 0g protein, 6g carbs, 0g fat)

- Toppings like mushrooms, onions, peppers (25 calories, 1g protein, 5g carbs, 0g fat per 1/2 cup)

- 2 Tbsp. shredded mozzarella (50 calories, 4g protein, 1g carbs, 4g fat)

- Directions: Top crust or flatbread with sauce, vegetables and cheese. Bake at 400F until crust is crisp and cheese melted.

Day 30 Totals: Calories - 1245, Protein - 77g, Carbs - 178g, Fat - 45g

Also, don't forget to drink plenty of water throughout the day!

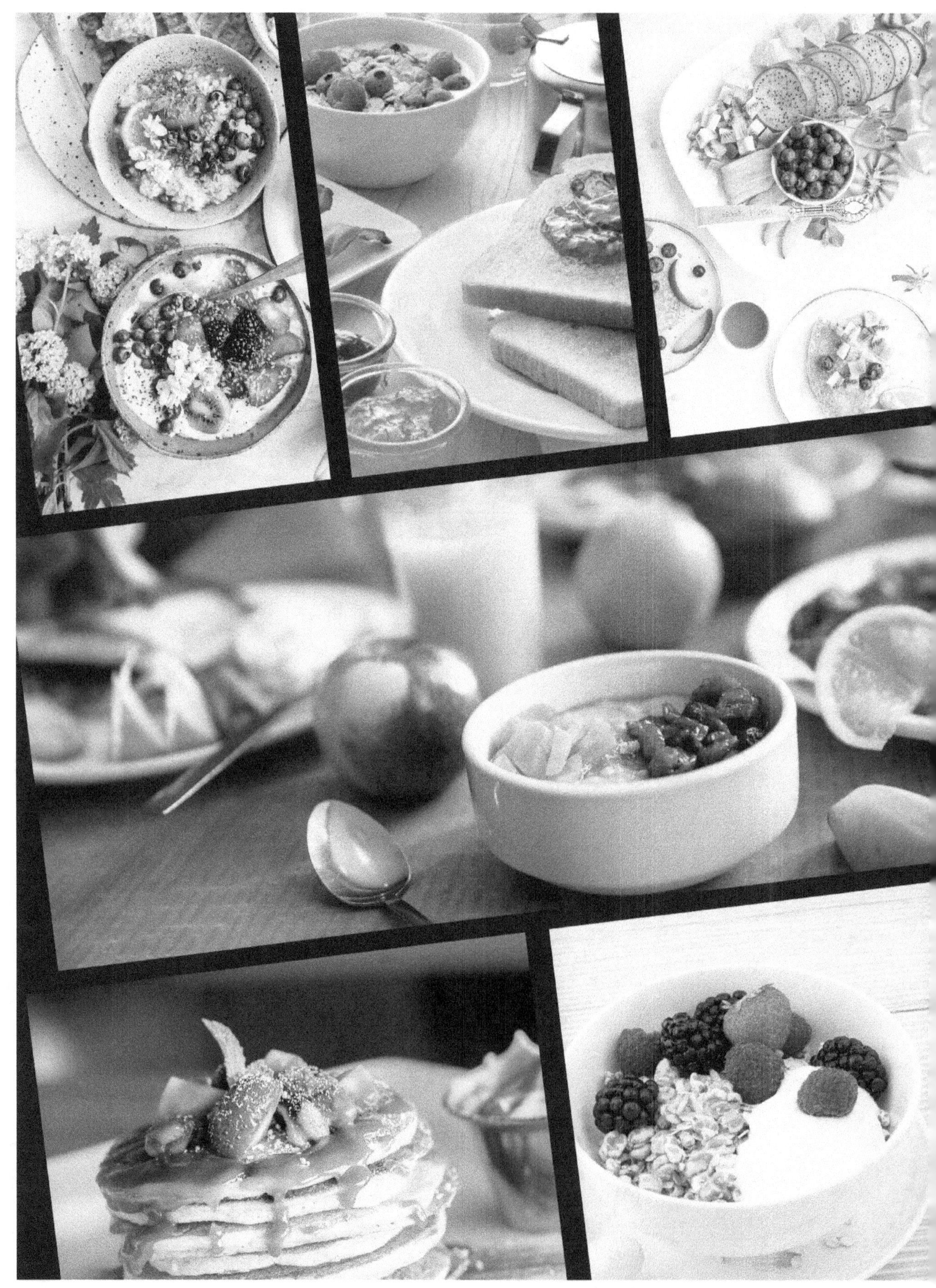

Master grocery list organized by category for the 30 day healthy meal plan:

Produce:

- Vegetables: spinach, lettuce (romaine, mixed greens), tomatoes (cherry, grape, plum), carrots, celery, bell peppers, onion, garlic, broccoli, cauliflower, green beans, potatoes, sweet potatoes, brussels sprouts, butternut squash, zucchini, mushrooms, kale, cucumber, avocado

- Fruits: lemons, limes, bananas, apples, berries (strawberries, blueberries, raspberries, blackberries), pineapple, grapes, acai packets

Proteins:

- Meat: chicken breast, turkey breast, lean ground turkey, flank steak, sirloin steak, pork tenderloin, pork chops, tilapia, cod, salmon

- Eggs and Dairy: eggs, shredded cheddar cheese, feta cheese, parmesan cheese, mozzarella cheese, plain Greek yogurt, cottage cheese, milk, almond milk

- Plant-based: tofu, canned tuna, canned salmon, canned chickpeas, black beans, edamame beans, lentils

Grains:

- Whole grains and flour: old fashioned oats, quinoa, brown rice, whole wheat pasta, corn tortillas, whole wheat tortillas, whole wheat bread, whole wheat pizza crust, whole wheat flatbread

Other:

- Herbs and Seasonings: garlic, onion, chia seeds, flaxseed, everything bagel seasoning, Cajun seasoning, Italian seasoning, cumin, chili powder, paprika, red pepper flakes, oregano, thyme, rosemary, curry powder, taco seasoning, sea salt, black pepper

- Oils and dressings: olive oil, sesame oil, balsamic vinegar, red wine vinegar, lemon juice, lime juice, honey mustard dressing, Caesar dressing, ranch dressing

- Sauces: soy sauce, salsa, marinara sauce, pesto, pizza sauce, hot sauce

- Sweeteners: maple syrup, honey

- Nuts, seeds and nut butters: walnuts, almonds, cashews, pecans, Brazil nuts, peanuts, natural peanut butter, natural almond butter, sunflower seed butter

- Condiments: mustard, mayonnaise, ketchup, relish, hummus, tahini

- Snacks and baking: granola, dried fruit, protein powder, frozen acai smoothie packs, applesauce, crackers, bread crumbs, dried lentils, canned beans, coconut milk

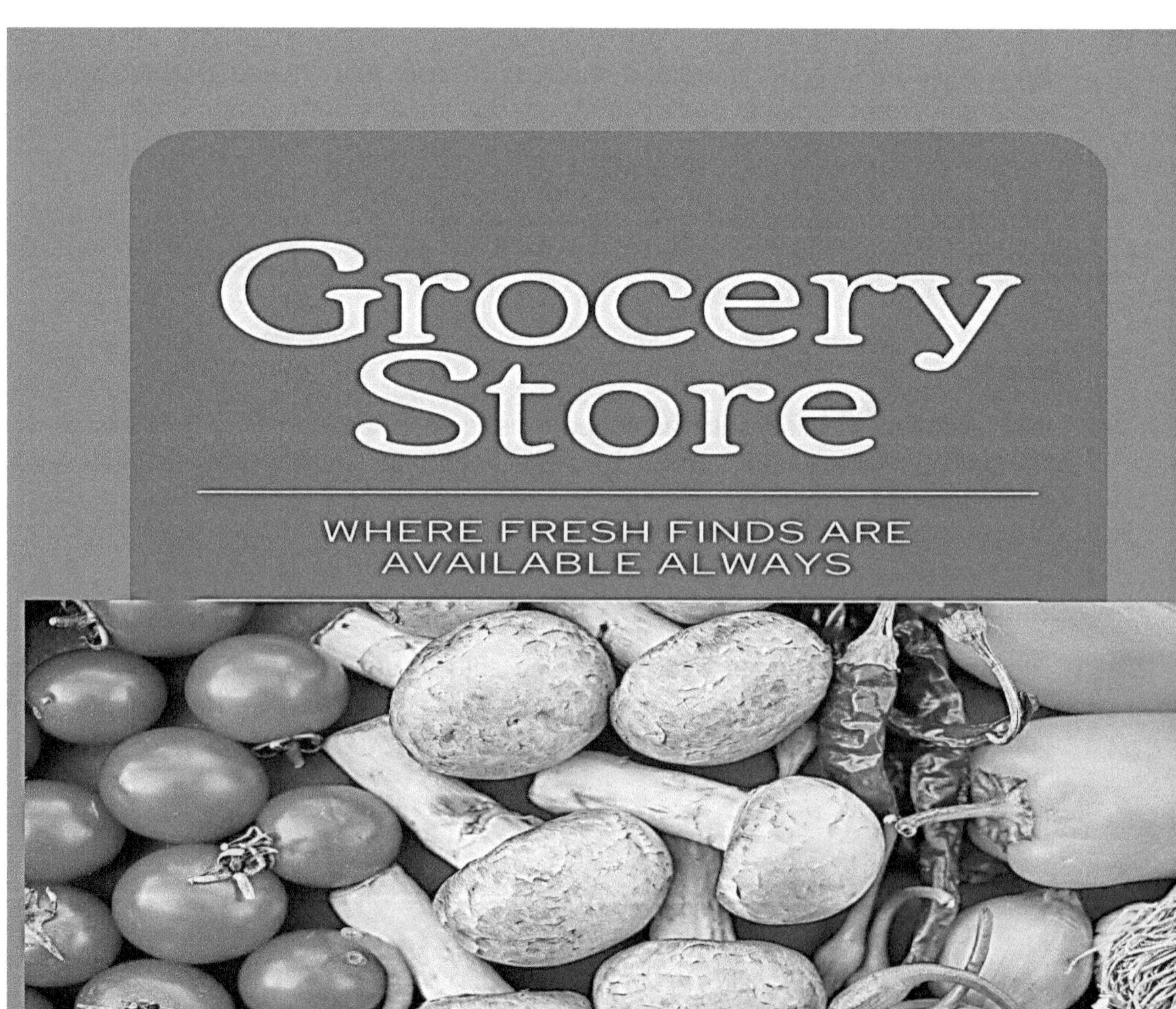

www.ingramcontent.com/pod-product-compliance
Lightning Source LLC
Chambersburg PA
CBHW080928260726
48661CB00010B/3841